TRANS PLANT ED

MY CYSTIC FIBROSIS DOUBLE-LUNG TRANSPLANT STORY

ALLISON WATSON

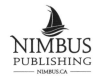

NIMBUS
PUBLISHING
— NIMBUS.CA —

Nimbus Publishing Limited
3660 Strawberry Hill Street, Halifax, NS, B3K 5A9
(902) 455-4286 nimbus.ca

Printed and bound in Canada
NB1358

Editor: Paula Sarson
Design: John van der Woude, JVDW Designs

Library and Archives Canada Cataloguing in Publication
Title: Transplanted : my cystic fibrosis double-lung transplant story / Allison Watson
Names: Watson, Allison, author.
Identifiers: Canadiana (print) 20189068310 | Canadiana (ebook) 20189068329 | ISBN 9781771087179 (softcover) | ISBN 9781771087186 (HTML)
Subjects: LCSH: Watson, Allison. | LCSH: Watson, Allison—Health. | LCSH: Cystic fibrosis—Patients—Canada—Biography. | LCSH: Lungs—Transplantation—Patients—Canada—Biography.
Classification: LCC RC858.C95 W38 2019 | DDC 362.1963/720092—dc23

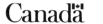 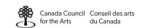

Nimbus Publishing acknowledges the financial support for its publishing activities from the Government of Canada, the Canada Council for the Arts, and from the Province of Nova Scotia. We are pleased to work in partnership with the Province of Nova Scotia to develop and promote our creative industries for the benefit of all Nova Scotians.

For my organ donor; thank you for saving my life.

DISCLAIMER

This is my transplant story as I remember it. I was heavily medicated for most of the important parts and may not remember all the events in chronological order. For the retelling of this story, I've relied on my blog posts and others' memories, the latter of which may not be entirely accurate as my family was doing their best to support me at the time instead of taking detailed notes for a future book.

I have done my best to describe medical terms and events, but I am not a medical professional. My view of procedures may be vastly different from that of a doctor or nurse. Dr. Internet can help provide examples in areas I have missed.

This book is not intended as medical advice! Do not treat it as such.

CONTENTS

PREFACE

I opened my eyes and everything was dark. I knew I was alone, in a hospital bed, but I wasn't sure on which wing or floor. I was pretty sure I was still in the Toronto General Hospital (TGH) but had no idea how much time had passed since I had last seen my family. When I tried to call out for a nurse, I found I couldn't speak due to a tube lodged in my throat. My arms felt as if they were weighed down with lead, so I couldn't wave for attention either. As I looked for a call bell to summon a nurse, I realized that I couldn't focus on anything: my vision was blurry and the world was spinning a little. My glasses were nowhere to be found. I could see people moving in the hallway, but they seemed to be spinning too. No one was coming into my room.

The dead silence was so unusual. No machines were beeping, no people were talking, none of the usual hospital noises.

Despite the lead feeling in my arms, I tried to wave in someone from the people milling about in the hallway, but no one was coming to check on me. They were all moving in jerky motions while I kept waving. I quickly exhausted myself and lay motionless, wondering what was happening.

I started to panic as I was suddenly positive the blurred vision and spinning world meant that I had carbon dioxide poisoning. I needed to tell someone what was wrong. My assumption wasn't such a stretch, as the last thing I remembered was being told that my carbon dioxide levels were high. I was sure I was either still in that hazy, poisoned world or that it was happening again. My panic mounted while I continued to be unable to get anyone into the room to help me. The people I kept seeing in the hallway were ignoring me. And why did the unit have a cardboard cut-out of a smiling, mustachioed man in a sombrero selling tacos?

Eventually, someone solidified in the doorway to tell me that I needed to wait for my nurse to return from her break. I tried to communicate to him through hand gestures that I was being poisoned, but he didn't understand my frantic waving. I must have somehow conveyed my panic, as he reluctantly stepped into the room. He brought in a paper and pencil and gave it to me so I could write down what I was trying to say. I grabbed them eagerly but discovered that my hands wouldn't respond to the motions I tried to make. Instead, they were shaking uncontrollably and my eyes couldn't focus enough on the paper to see what I was attempting to write. In my frustration, I wrote a bunch of squiggly lines and handed the paper back to the man.

He then summoned someone else into the room to try to decipher my scrawl, but this woman was just as befuddled as he was. After many, many tries, I managed to write "CO_2," and they seemed to get the point that I thought my levels were high. The woman hung a bag of something on my IV pole and I felt a bit better. (For all I know, it was just stronger pain or sleep medication.) The man then asked if he could pray over me, to which I didn't respond as I was still confused, though certain I was poisoned. He prayed and then left the room. I soon fell back asleep.

When I woke up again, lights were on and there was a nurse sitting behind the glass panel in front of my room. She noticed I was awake and came into the room, apologized for the other man's behaviour and that I had wakened alone. I gestured to my throat and the equipment in the room by way of asking why it was there and what had happened.

She responded, "Need a suction?"

I had no idea what she meant, but I must've nodded as she suddenly began shoving a tube into my lungs. It felt like I was choking and made me want to cough but when I tried, it was impossible. I didn't have the energy to move the muscles required to cough. As quickly as it had started, the suctioning was over and the tube was gone. I could breathe easier, but I still had no idea what had just happened.

All the nurse told me was that it was still early and I needed to try to go back to sleep. The next time I wakened, a different nurse told me that physiotherapy would be in later that day to get me up. I gestured to convey all my questions, so she brought me a pen and paper to write again. I tried to write down my multitude of questions such as, "Where am I?" and, "Do I have carbon dioxide poisoning?" but my hands were still too shaky and my eyes still couldn't focus. Somehow, the nurse realized that I was panicking and told me I was experiencing side effects from the medication. I wasn't sure what medication she was referring to but was happy to know, at last, that I wasn't being poisoned.

About the fourth time I woke up, I finally managed to communicate to the nurse that I had no idea what had happened. Where was I? Did I have a lung transplant? Was it good news? I don't remember much from those days, but I do remember her staring at me and saying, "Oh honey, yes, it's good news, very good news. You had your lung transplant four days ago."

PART I

PRE-TRANSPLANT

MY LIFE UNTIL
OCTOBER 2013

1

PREPPING FOR TRANSPLANT

A HARD SHIFT TO MAKE

I grew up knowing that I had cystic fibrosis (CF). Having a chronic illness is hard to hide from children when they have to take pills before every meal and do aerosol masks. Besides the clinic appointments every three months, daily aerosol masks and chest percussions, and being required to eat chips every night for the extra calories, I had a fairly normal childhood.

As a December baby, I was the smallest in my class at school; New Brunswick, where we lived at the time, went by the calendar year for classroom placements. My parents debated keeping me in kindergarten another year to give me a chance to catch up, but by that time, I had a group of close friends with whom I wanted to stay for grade one. Having CF didn't affect my friendships, and although everyone knew I had it, the only difference about my school experience compared to theirs was that I had to go to the office every recess for a nutritional drink called Ensure for extra calories. Dad always did presentations for the school at the start of the year to explain CF and fundraise through the Zellers CF Moonwalk (now called the Walk to Make Cystic Fibrosis History). My friends understood why I had to do aerosol masks during sleepovers and why I took so many pills with each meal. We didn't talk about it, and it wasn't a big factor in my life growing up.

Living with CF was part of our lives—my older sister, Amy, has it too—but it was not something that defined us. Our parents never let us use having CF as an excuse to get out of anything, and I think having each other reinforced the idea that we were not special because we had a disability. I use the word *disability* in relation to CF and while other people may not like the word for themselves, I feel it is accurate for me. While having CF may not have been causing me disablement when I was younger, it still limited my life in some ways. Although I did my best not to be defined by having CF, it would be naïve for me to say that it did not affect my life in any way.

I was hospitalized quite often as a toddler but Amy and I were both relatively healthy as children. We were only hospitalized once in our teens for two weeks for what we called a "tune-up." It was a relatively easy hospitalization as well. We went to the IWK clinic, thinking only I would be hospitalized, but it turned out Amy was faring much worse than I was. My health was improved but they stuck me in the hospital anyway, "since Amy was there." I guess the doctors figured it was all the same to my parents if they had one or two children in the hospital, not that I remain bitter to this day about Amy causing me to be hospitalized. It was actually fine: we spent two weeks getting IV antibiotics, playing Yahtzee in the hospital's family room, and annoying the physiotherapist because we wouldn't stay in our room so we often missed our physiotherapy time. Those things, and a cute volunteer named Josh who gave us a Calvin and Hobbes book when we left, are about all I remember from those two weeks.

As I've grown older, I've realized what a huge blessing it has been to have a sister with the same disease. I know that's weird to say. I should want her to be healthy. And it's not like I want her to have a fatal disease. It's just that it has been helpful to have someone to talk to who's had the same experiences as me.

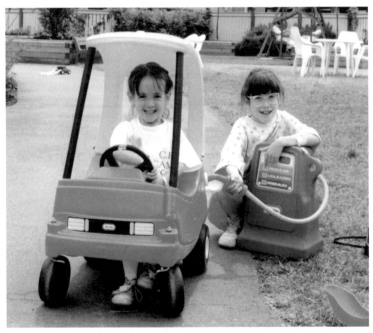

Allison (left) and her sister, Amy, at the IWK Health Centre play-park in 1991 during a hospitalization. Allison was admitted frequently as a young child due to her failure to gain weight. (Donna Watson)

I could complain to her when I had stomach cramps and she wouldn't panic and tell me to go to the hospital; instead, she would make comments like, "That sucks," or, "Maybe you forgot to take your digestive enzymes." I think that we pushed each other, even if we didn't realize it at the time. I mean, if she could hike for an hour, so could I. There was no reason for me not to do anything, because there she was with the same disability as me, so who was I to complain. Of course there were times when it would have been better to stop and let our bodies rest, so in that regard we occasionally pushed ourselves too far—more so as we got older and our lungs started to decline.

It's hard to know where the line is. Having CF means that you spend many days simply pushing yourself to get out of bed in the morning. It can be a struggle to do "simple" tasks like showering or cooking supper. And then when you want to go out with friends or go for a bike ride, it can be even more exhausting. Once I reached my twenties, if I had stopped doing activities because I felt tired or short of breath, I would have rarely left the house. And rarely leaving the house starts the downward spiral of feeling worse, which leads to never leaving the house, which leads to feeling worse…and so on. It's a terrible cycle.

I've always known that having CF meant having a shortened life expectancy. But knowing the facts while healthy is different from having a doctor suddenly tell you that your options are to die in one to three years or take a chance with a lung transplant. Some people with CF have traumatic stories about the first time they realized they were born with a life-shortening illness. I don't have that story. I feel like I always knew, though I must have learned it at some point, either at the CF clinic or from Amy. According to our parents, Amy found out when our cousin told her, "You'll never graduate from high school because you're going to die early." However, Amy doesn't remember that happening, so clearly she wasn't traumatized either.

I realize it can be scary for children to learn they won't live as long as their friends. But while we were growing up, that was not how we thought about it. Our parents were more focused on what we would do with the time we had. There was no point in thinking about a shortened lifespan when we could focus on the present. Why spend the time you have worrying about a future that may never come? I think it also helped that I was fairly healthy through high school, so I didn't feel as though I was being "left behind." I filled out university applications and dreamed of a career along with the rest of my friends. The only real difference was that I laughed when anyone mentioned pensions or retirement planning. Because I had spent so little time in the hospital, dying and being acutely sick were abstract concepts.

The first time I found it emotionally difficult to have a shortened life expectancy was on my twentieth birthday. It hit me then that I had reached the halfway mark of my predicted lifespan. It wasn't the best time to be sad and pouty because my family was spending a week of the school Christmas break in the Bahamas. We were vacationing at the home of a missionary couple who were spending the week back in the United States; we couldn't pass up the opportunity of having a place to stay in the Caribbean. Although we almost didn't get into the country because Mom and Dad weren't prepared for customs questions such as, "Who are you staying with?" and "What is the house address?" Their responses of, "With friends we've never met," and, "The address is written on a piece of paper in the car they left in the parking lot for us, and the keys are in the dash," were not the answers border security wanted to hear.

Somehow, they did let us into the country and we enjoyed our first-ever Christmas on the beach. It was a great vacation, and we were thrilled to have our first Christmas away from home. Amy, who was working as a nurse in neonatal intensive care at the time, couldn't come with us because nurses have the worst work schedules; she called us, envious, while we were enjoying Christmas Day and she was getting pooped on by babies. Despite the pleasant Christmas, however, on my twentieth birthday a few days later, I was feeling gloomy because I had possibly reached "my halfway point."

I knew that there was no guarantee I would live until I was forty or that I would die the day I turned forty, but on that birthday I mourned everything that I would miss. It is hard to describe what I was feeling at that moment. It was essentially that I was too old to have accomplished so little, and that I was not going to have enough time to fit in everything I wanted from life in the mere twenty years I had left. In retrospect, I realize how ridiculous I was behaving, but I also think it was important for me to process these thoughts at the time. I think realizing that I wouldn't be able to save adventures and trips for after I retired meant that I was more adventurous in my twenties than I might otherwise have been.

Just as I grew up knowing that I had a fatal disease, I also knew that one day I might need a lung transplant. In the '90s, a lung transplant was still considered a new medical procedure: the first one done on a person with CF was in 1988. It was a medical breakthrough for the CF community that was starting to be discussed as a possibility as an end-of-life treatment. Nonetheless, growing up, the idea was so abstract that it held no real meaning or fear. My family would often talk about it as something that both Amy and I would probably one day need. We would joke casually about "when I need new lungs," or, "I hope this isn't the infection that requires me to need new lungs."

Even with my awareness that I might one day require and be eligible for a transplant, it didn't make it any easier to accept when the day arrived. When the doctor first mentioned starting the workup process for a lung transplant, I burst into tears and refused to talk about it. I was in denial about how sick I was and didn't want to accept that I had reached the point of needing a transplant. I had had a string of infections over a few years—several that required hospitalization with strong IV antibiotics—so I knew my lungs were not doing well, but I could not believe I was at the point of needing new ones. They only do that to people who have a life expectancy of less than three years. I couldn't be at that point. Could I?

I felt as though I had failed myself by needing a transplant before Amy. As she was the older sister, I thought she should have to go first. I also struggled with the fact that even though she was the older sibling, she was doing much better than me health-wise. I conveniently forgot that she never seemed to get as many lung infections as me, bounced back from infections quicker, and was healthier overall. It took getting pneumonia twice in one year, and a long hospital stay, before I started to admit that I was going to need a transplant.

In fact, when I had pneumonia and was subsequently hospitalized in November 2012, that was the first time I had the physical feeling that I was dying. It made me panicked and slightly depressed. I had no energy, threw up all the time, and had a lot of back pain. It was terrifying to be that ill.

After that hospitalization, I somehow convinced the doctor to let me return to work, even though she was quite reluctant. I was not yet ready to concede that I needed to stop. It was a hard winter, and I struggled at work and at home. Working took up all of my energy, so I would spend my time off in a state of near-exhaustion, recovering. I was in a cycle that couldn't last forever, but I wanted it to last as long as possible. I knew that as soon as I stopped, I would not be returning to work any time soon.

During that time, I was fortunate that I had access to my workplace's mental health program. It gave employees access to counsellors either by phone, email, or in face-to-face meetings. I opted for the email route because I found I could express myself better through writing. I also found that it helped me work through my emotions when I had to think about what to write, put it down coherently, and reread the text to make sure it made sense to someone else. The counsellor was remarkably helpful as I worked through a lot of my anxieties around needing a lung transplant and dealing with death. She had me do exercises about my fears and gave me a lot of questions to ponder. When I was anxious that I was becoming depressed, she helped me realize that it was normal to feel sad and hopeless when encountering something in life of such great magnitude.

I made it through most of the winter feeling tired, coughing more than usual, being short of breath, but overall persevering. I tried to hide my exhaustion at the hospital where I worked as a recreational therapist. It became increasingly difficult as nurses would hear me coughing up phlegm in the bathroom, and patients would wonder about my shortness of breath. I tried to pass it off as a cold, but this also became harder as the months progressed. I just didn't have the energy anymore to get through the workday cycle.

At the time, I was organizing a two-week trip to visit my brother, David, who was living in Spain. I love planning trips and travelling, so researching beaches on the Canary Islands was a great distraction. Then my cough increased to even scarier-than-normal levels, my appetite plummeted, and I started throwing up massive amounts of phlegm. My back hurt, I struggled to stand up while showering, and found it painful to breathe deeply. I had pneumonia again. It was all over.

I went to the local hospital for an x-ray. As soon as the results were available, the Halifax CF nurse called and told me to "get here now with an overnight bag." When I arrived to see the team, the doctor immediately pulled me off work "for the foreseeable future," and told me if I went to Spain, I would return in a body bag. She was not one to beat around the bush. Instead of going to Europe and having a fun vacation, I ended up in the hospital. Testing for a lung transplant began in full force.

There are only five transplant clinics in Canada—none in Atlantic Canada—so all patients from the Halifax clinic are assessed by the Toronto transplant team. If approved for a transplant, the patient must move to Toronto to wait, as the transplant team requires the person to be living within a two-and-a-half-hour drive of the hospital.

One of the common misconceptions about lung transplants is that every person with CF will eventually get the chance to have one. While hospitals are performing more and more lung transplants every year, it's still not a viable option for everyone. There are many factors that make a person ineligible, and the teams are rather strict about whom they will allow. There is such a limited number of donor lungs that they need to make sure recipients have the best possible chance of succeeding with the lungs available. Also, a lung transplant is done as an end-stage procedure for people with CF, so a person has to be quite ill, but not so sick that they can't recover from the surgery.

Generally, the criteria is that a person's forced expiratory volume in one second (FEV1) has to be less than 30% of the predicted output for someone of their age and weight. Once a person's FEV1 drops below 30%, statistically, they have a life expectancy of one to three years and are now considered eligible for the end-stage procedure. Having pneumonia dropped my FEV1 to a new low of 22%, and while it did jump back up to 28% after the hospitalization, the increase was mostly due to the strong antibiotics pulsing through my veins.

The other criterion to be accepted into the transplant program is that the other organs have to be functioning as well as possible. People with CF tend to have weak hearts due to the fact that our hearts struggle to make up for lung deficiencies. While the lungs attempt to get air in and out, the rest of the body struggles to keep everything running. The kidneys and liver can also be weakened for people with CF as years of medication and antibiotics tend to stress any organ trying to keep toxins out of the body. Post-transplant medications are especially hard on the kidneys and liver, so doctors need to make sure that everything is as healthy as possible before dumping even more medication in.

During my hospitalization in February 2013, I completed a lot of the pre-transplant workup. I did a six-minute walk test, an x-ray, CT scan, and massive amounts of blood work. I was discharged back home after three weeks of antibiotics and waited to hear from the overlords in Toronto as to whether or not I would qualify to move on to the next stage of testing. It was an anxious few months. It seemed as though I was testing to qualify for a game I didn't want to play. Will I be too healthy? Will I be too sick? Will my liver be damaged from that one night I drank too much? The Halifax doctors basically told me that I could be denied for any reason: being too healthy or too sick, having something else wrong with me, not checking my blood sugar levels every day, looking at them the wrong way...well, you get the idea.

As I had been pumped full of antibiotics, my lung function jumped up by 10%. This was great for my health and showed that I had responded well to the antibiotics, but then the doctor mentioned that my lung function may have improved too much for a transplant. Nonetheless, she told me that "we should probably still go ahead with the process." I agreed, thinking, "Of course you should go ahead with the process. Two weeks ago you were panicking that catching a cold would be the death of me and now I'm suddenly good to go?" I was baffled. In the end, I was just on a medication high; once the medication was out of my system, my lung function returned to almost where it had been before I got pneumonia.

There is an effect that Amy and I like to call the "antibiotic high," which is the feeling we get after being hospitalized. We feel 100% better after being pumped full of antibiotics for two or three weeks, as the medication suppresses any cough, phlegm production, and shortness of breath. Our lung functions jump up for a while, and we feel ready to take on anything. However, after about a week off the medication, when the antibiotics wear off, we go back to feeling as we did before we went into the hospital—only, hopefully, a few percentage points better. Thankfully, at the time, I managed to hang on to the antibiotic high and didn't crash back down to 22% until over a year after that hospitalization. Although I was still ill during that time, I was not declining rapidly and was perceived as stable enough to be able to wait in Toronto for lungs as well as to survive the actual operation. I was in the sweet spot of being sick but not too sick.

Waiting for the results of transplant testing is a mind game. Like I've said, you have to be sick enough to require the transplant but healthy enough to survive the surgery and rehabilitation. You also have to not have anything else wrong with you and be mentally prepared for the trauma that comes with the surgery and recovery. Providing you aren't rejected, you move to Toronto to wait for the surgery and are started on an intense physiotherapy program. Sometimes, because of all the exercise during physiotherapy, people show an improvement in their lung function, causing them to become "too healthy" for a transplant. Then they have to wait until their lung function drops—but of course, it can't drop too low because then they wouldn't have the ability to survive the surgery. People continue to play the "transplant game," trying to stay in the elusive zone between being too healthy and being terminally ill, all while trying to be perfect patients so one day they might win, maybe, a new set of lungs.

I understand why the majority of people listed for transplant are on anti-anxiety medication. The process causes a lot of stress. While I waited, I started having trouble sleeping—not that I had been sleeping well before the testing, due to all my coughing and needing to be propped up on three pillows to make breathing easier. Now, in addition to that, the "what if" game was keeping me up. Instead of taking sleep medication that tended to give me nightmares or left me feeling groggy in the morning, I started listening to podcasts to lull me to sleep.

One immediate outcome from all the testing I had to undergo was that my six-minute walk test showed I needed to be using oxygen while exercising. Even with all my obvious health problems, I was not mentally ready for that step. To me, requiring oxygen meant that this was the end of my life, and, less dramatically, the end of being able to do anything I enjoyed. Once I started using oxygen to help me breathe, there was no going back, and it was a visible reminder that I was dying.

During my recreation therapy internship at a nursing home for my recreation therapy degree, I had been surprised to find myself uncomfortable around the people who required oxygen. I kept trying to shake off the discomfort and found that it was the people who required oxygen and were bedridden who distressed me more than those who used oxygen but were still mobile and active. The few people who were bedridden on oxygen were usually frail, and they were a stark reminder that one day that would probably be me, only at a much younger age. I felt as though I was being shown my future, and it terrified me.

I remained in denial for a long time about requiring oxygen, even though the team told me I needed it only "upon exertion," which is often the first step for a person in lung decline. The idea is that since the body is limited by being unable to breathe, if that person wears oxygen, the body will not struggle as much and can therefore exercise harder and longer. The more we exercise, the stronger we become and the easier it is to breathe. It does not necessarily help improve lung function, but it does help strengthen the muscles around the lungs, making the body healthier overall.

Another problem with being prescribed oxygen to wear "upon exertion" was, at that time, most activities were exhausting for me. I was self-conscious wearing it in public, so while I would strap it on at home to lift weights or stretch, I did not like using it around other people. As I had been strongly encouraged to start exercising regularly, I signed up for the local gym but was too nervous carrying in my oxygen. Consequently, I wasn't able to do much. I would walk slowly on the treadmill, which, while better than nothing, was not as helpful as it could have been. Afterward I would use oxygen to help recover, but it was not quite the same. I became less self-conscious as time went on, and once winter was over, I put the tanks in my bike panniers while cycling or I would throw one in a backpack the few times Isaiah, my partner, and I went on short hikes. I still refused to wear oxygen in public as I felt it would be an obvious sign that I was ill, and I hated that idea.

✦

During the months I waited to hear from the team in Toronto, I did feel okay physically; I was no longer acutely sick. The regular exercise seemed to help and my lungs were holding steady with a FEV1 of 26%. However, I thought a lot about death and dying and what it would be like to die. I wasn't as panicked as

I had been back in November, but I was still scared overall. I admit that I spent a lot of time crying in the bathroom about what would happen if I didn't get the transplant, what would happen if I did get the transplant, or what would happen if I went for the transplant and it didn't happen. It wasn't a continuous feeling of anxiety but rather something that would hit me from time to time in quiet moments. To work through these feelings, I would cry for a short spell and then carry on with life.

As a way to deal with my emotions, I turned to my support system and had a lot of fascinating conversations with my friends about life, death, dying, and post-death. Some people were uncomfortable talking about death with me but most seemed to know that I just needed someone to listen while I worked through my fears. I know some people feel as though it's morbid to talk about death, but this was my coping strategy. If I was going to die, I was going to die well-informed and have the best possible death. I figured we, as a society, spend so much time planning and thinking about what happens when someone comes into the world, we should spend at least *some* time figuring out what to do when a person leaves. The more I read blogs about dying and what happens to an actual corpse, the more comfortable I became. It was much more cathartic for me to learn as much as I could about the situation than to deny its possibility. And I could no longer deny the fact that I was not getting better.

In April 2013 I learned that I had passed the initial round of testing and was due to be in Toronto during the second week of July for round two. At that point, I still didn't know if I even wanted to have the transplant, but I knew that I had to at least do the testing to see if I would be accepted.

While I waited for July to arrive, Isaiah and I spent a few days camping and biking on Prince Edward Island in early June. I made it out for a few short rides, but spent most of the time reading on the beach, waiting for him to be done. I forced myself to wear oxygen while biking and became less self-conscious about it. I realized that if I didn't wear it, I wouldn't be able to do anything. I lectured myself that I needed to check my pride and get on with my life. There was no point sitting around pining for what I wished was happening when I could be living within the parameters of my new reality. The few days on the Island finally hammered home to me that if I didn't do what I could with what I had, then I would be both missing out and miserable. This was the reality check I needed: I might as well embrace what health I had while I still had it.

My entire family loves to travel. I'm not sure where this comes from. Maybe it all began when Mom and Dad packed up the van and drove us all across the country when we were young, or maybe it's from being raised with the attitude to take opportunities when they come because we may never get the chance again. Amy and I may have shortened life expectancies, but we never let CF stop us from doing what we wanted: as long as we were healthy enough, we were going to travel.

So after my Prince Edward Island vacation, Amy convinced me—it did not take much—to take a road trip to Newfoundland in late June 2013 as an escape from my thoughts and from my apartment. It was a much needed vacation. We drove all over Newfoundland, seeing whales and puffins, chasing icebergs, and camping in the rain. We drove to St. John's, ducked down to visit St. Pierre and Miquelon, went back across the island, up to St. Anthony, and eventually back down to Gros Morne National Park. The struggles of travelling with a disability were much more evident during our trip to Newfoundland than they had been during any previous vacations.

As CF is a hidden disease, other people often have a hard time recognizing our level of illness. To them, Amy and I look perfectly healthy. The downside to having a hidden disability is that people make assumptions about your abilities. Normally, that would be something I embrace, as people don't automatically assume limitations before getting to know me. However, it worked against Amy and me when we got to the island of St. Pierre. When we arrived from the ferry, we immediately went to the tourist information centre to get a map along with some information on the island. We had planned on taking a taxi to our B&B because it was outside the main touristy area, and atop a giant hill. Since the ferry was "pedestrian only," we had assumed there would be cabs waiting when we got off to take people to their hotels. We should have known better than to assume anything while travelling to a new place, but we had not yet learned our lesson.

We asked the worker at the information centre where we could get a cab. He proceeded to tell us that "Young healthy girls like you can walk there, no problem!" He outlined on the map the route to take, ignoring our insistence that we would indeed like to take a cab. Our French was not strong enough to argue with the young Frenchman, so, annoyed, we went to the bank to get some euros and returned to the tourist centre, hoping he would be gone. Thankfully, he was. The friendly woman working at the desk called us a cab, only after asking several times if we were sure we didn't want to walk.

Amy wanted to tell them that I was actually carrying a tank of oxygen in my backpack, so, *Yes, we're sure we don't want to walk*. However, arguing in a second language is challenging, so we just kept insisting that we would like a cab. Eventually one arrived. During the first minute of the ride, I wondered if maybe we could have walked after all. The second minute, I was happy we were in a car as the hill suddenly became crazy steep. It was a short distance but not worth struggling up. Later, we walked down the hill to tour the town and had no trouble getting a cab after our supper of crepes by the wharf. Apparently, when it's dark and raining, people are not as insistent that you walk.

For our last few days in Newfoundland, we camped in Gros Morne National Park, did the fjord tour, drove around looking for caribou, and tried to do a little hike. That hike turned out to be a horrible decision. It was humid that day, and I was labouring to breathe. The hike was flat along the bottom of a ridge, so I didn't think it would be difficult, but I struggled the entire time. It was one of the first times in my life where I wasn't able to push through an inability to breathe and keep going.

Of course, I hadn't been able to do certain activities in the past. But mostly I would avoid ventures that I knew I wouldn't be able to do, and for the ones that ended up being borderline, I would take breaks and keep on going. For example, when we were on vacation in Greece, on one of the islands we hiked to see "Zeus's cave." I struggled up the hill to that site—I needed constant breaks, threw up a bit, and took many puffers—but I was able to make it to the cave. It was one of the borderline activities that I thought I could do, probably shouldn't have, but kept going anyway.

In Newfoundland that day with my sister, I just couldn't do it. I couldn't walk anymore in the heat and humidity. We had to turn back, and even then, I had to stop a lot and stick my feet in the streams to cool off. That aborted hike marked a low point in my life. I had to make a significant mental adjustment, finally realizing that what I thought I could do and what I could actually do were two very different things. I was a long time admitting to myself that I was seriously ill. Even though I had always had a chronic disease, it was a hard shift to make.

2

TESTING IN TORONTO, TESTING OF PATIENCE

The second week of July 2013 arrived quickly. It was time to fly to Toronto for my week of pre-transplant assessment. I struggled emotionally the week before the departure. I didn't know if I was making the right decision and I was terrified of what would happen in Toronto. I had been sent the Almighty Transplant Manual, which was supposed to explain the entire assessment process. It helped, but so much seemed like a great unknown.

The morning we were to fly out, I had a full-blown panic attack in the bathroom. I told Isaiah that I wasn't going or ever leaving the bathroom. He would have to call everyone to cancel everything; the bathroom would be my new home. He eventually talked me out of the bathroom and convinced me to go to the airport. The situation was becoming way too real. I was not prepared to be another step closer to the actual transplant; I had to emotionally adjust with every step. It's much easier to cope with the idea: "I might get a transplant," or: "In a week, I'll go to Toronto," than with the reality of getting on the plane.

My coping mechanism was to freak out as much as I felt was needed and then try to find a way to distract myself until I could process the intensity of my emotions. My distraction during the actual flight was that none of the flight attendants seemed as if they had ever used oxygen on a plane before and had no idea how to set it up. They all consulted on how to set up the tank. Once they eventually got it going, they checked about every twenty minutes that it was still running. I'm sure they all had a training day on oxygen tanks at some point but had not recently put it into practice. It's fun to be a guinea pig sometimes.

The week-long assessment in Toronto involved many tests and meetings with various people from the pre-transplant team. We stayed at a cute B&B close to the hospital, which made the commute back and forth easy. The greater stress was figuring out where all the different appointments were once we were in the hospital. It seemed overwhelmingly large, all the wings and elevators had different names, and we always felt like we were late for the appointments. Of course, by the time I left Toronto, I would know that hospital much better than anyone ought to.

On Monday morning I had fasting blood work, an electrocardiogram, and an x-ray at the TGH—all fairly standard. The most stressful part was when a scary nurse demanded that I give her a sputum sample. I informed her that I, miraculously, hadn't been coughing up anything lately and asked if it would be possible to do a throat swab instead like they did at the Halifax clinic. She responded that it wasn't possible and I needed to go into the bathroom and cough something up. I gave it my best shot. I coughed for a solid five minutes but nothing came up. I returned empty-handed and exhausted, only for her to ask if I had done it right and then "remind me" of how to cough up sputum.

In that moment, I wanted to slap her and every other health professional who has ever lectured a patient on the proper way to do a task they have done their entire lives. Of course I didn't, because people who slap nurses do not get new lungs. Instead, I patiently responded that I had done my best but I couldn't produce anything, and that there wasn't much more I could do. She told me that I wasn't allowed to eat anything until I could produce something, as food would compromise the sample. I was starving, and being told that I couldn't eat until I did something that I couldn't physically do was infuriating, especially since I had just read in the Almighty Transplant Manual that "It's OK if you can't produce a sample; many patients are unable to cough anything up." It did not say that I was not allowed to eat until I gave them something. I ended up taking the bottle back to the B&B with me, promising to return it "on the chance that I coughed something up." I never did. It was not a good start to the week. I was terrified that everyone in the system was going to be equally intimidating, lecturing me if I couldn't do what they wanted.

Tuesday was my day at the CF clinic at St. Michael's Hospital (St. Mike's). The CF team there wanted to meet me and do their own tests for their records. Even though St. Mike's is only a few blocks from the TGH, they could never seem to organize their records so that information could be shared. Theoretically, this information was supposed to be uploaded to a special server that everyone could access, but the staff rarely uploaded the information. As a result, it meant that I had to do everything for a second time at that hospital: another round of blood work, x-rays, and another sputum sample. Thankfully, that nurse said it was normal for people to be unable to cough up a sample because the antibiotics they are on tend to suppress production. She seemed horrified when I told her about the nurse at the TGH and said that she hoped that incident didn't give me a bad impression of health-care services in Toronto.

Everyone at St. Mike's was helpful and informative. They noticed that I was stressed to the max and tried to ease my fears. I did a set of lung function tests with them and my FEV1 came back at 48%! When I saw that on the screen during the test, I told the technician there must be some mistake. He dismissed my concerns, saying that perhaps Halifax used a different calculation and that every system was different. I kept saying it was wrong, but we continued with the tests. When the doctor came around for the assessment, he said that it was good I was doing the workup but he wasn't sure why they had sent me so early because my lung function was too high to be eligible for a transplant. I assured him that I was eligible, that my testing was wrong, and my lung function didn't spike to 48% in the past month. I surely would've noticed if I suddenly had a dramatic increase in lung function.

I kept insisting that the number was wrong until, finally, he looked at the information more closely. He noticed that my birthday had been entered so that the algorithm was set for someone who was eighty-six instead of twenty-six years old. The technician must've typed in my birth year instead of my age. If I had been eighty-six years old, it would've been good news because then I would've had 48% of the expected lung function. Unfortunately, I was still only twenty-six, so when adjusted properly, the calculation changed my FEV1 to be about 27% of the expected lung function for my age and body size. The doctor concluded that I was indeed eligible for a transplant.

Wednesday of that week was an easy day. I had an echocardiogram and the RNA MUGA test. This was all to make sure that my heart and liver were working smoothly. Isaiah bailed on me that day, and he managed to do some sightseeing in the city. The only sightseeing I did that week was at the restaurants on the street of our B&B and at the Art Gallery of Ontario, which was conveniently nearby and free that night.

Thursday was hard emotionally. I met with the pre-transplant coordinator as well as the social worker. The social worker made it clear that I needed to make up my mind about whether or not I wanted to be listed. The team doesn't like going through the entire process only to have someone back out, so she does interviews to gauge a candidate's emotional stability and ability to deal with the situation overall. She asked about my support systems, both emotional and financial. I told her that I had a great support system and there was no need to worry.

She mentioned that many people require anti-anxiety medication as the entire situation is anxiety inducing. She asked if I thought I needed some. I declined the medication at that time but said I would let her know if anything changed. She seemed slightly concerned for me because I almost burst into tears every time she asked how I was doing emotionally and whether I felt prepared to be listed. Truthfully, I was not doing well, but I couldn't express anything other than how terrifying the entire process seemed and how I didn't want to be sick.

There were many questions from the social worker and the pre-transplant coordinator about reflecting on my life at the moment as compared to the previous three weeks, six months, or year. I found those questions hard to answer. I'm not one to sit around and reflect on my life enough to know the answers. They also asked me about what I was able to do around the house at the moment compared to the previous year. I could answer that question, as it was more specific. I was able to say that not much had changed: I still did the same rough number of household chores but at a slightly slower rate and with more breaks.

Friday was much less exhausting, both emotionally and physically. My last test was an abdominal ultrasound which was less pleasant than I had anticipated. I envisioned it as a quick scan on my stomach, much like I've seen done on TV with pregnant women. Instead, it was more like being jabbed forcefully over and over again with the wand in and around my entire ribcage for about an hour. I did not get to nap as I had hoped. By the end of the day, I felt as though every part of me had been scrutinized to the fullest extent. If anything was wrong with me, they were going to find it.

Looking back, I know I made the right decision, but at the time, having to make the official decision was the most terrifying thing I had ever done. I was still not fully committed to the idea of going through with the transplant, yet I had to start thinking about what I was going to do if they said I was eligible. Up until that point, I had just been floating through the process, more passively going through the steps than making active decisions for myself. I kept telling myself that I could stop the process at any time, which helped me make the decisions to go forward with the testing. However, I was reaching the point of no return. Clearly, if I agreed to be listed and then moved to Toronto, it was not as though they could force me to do the transplant if I did change my mind. But I still needed to say yes or no to the move. I know that most people felt it should be a clear yes and that I would be crazy to not go through with it.

Yet, there was so much to consider. It's hard to study how much a lung transplant will extend a person's life as there is no do-over: you can't know what would've happened if the person hadn't had a transplant. Statistically, a person has one to three years to live once their lung function drops below 30% of the expected value, but I know of people who have lived five years at that number. So just because a doctor says you might die soon, doesn't mean you will.

The next day, Saturday, I felt much better and was ready for our flight home. I learned to compartmentalize my emotions and to push them away when other people were around. This practice also came in handy when later dealing with my lung transplant–related emotions; in other words, it helped me to not break into tears every five seconds.

After the intense week in Toronto, I was sent home to wait to hear if I would be accepted into the lung transplant program. It was a long month and a half of waiting. I tried to distract myself by taking care of my container garden, reading, going on short bike rides, learning how to knit, and visiting friends and family. The distractions mostly worked, but I still had moments of panic. Coming to terms with the fact that I was so sick and wouldn't be recovering any time in the near future continued to be a struggle.

Eventually, in the third week of August, while cottaging with my family on Prince Edward Island, I got the much-anticipated/much-dreaded phone call from Toronto. The pre-transplant coordinator told me that all my tests looked good. I was accepted into the program. I would like to say that a weight was lifted off my shoulders with that news, but it felt more as though I had been loaded down with more to inundate me. While there was some satisfaction that I could finally start planning my life beyond more than a month at a time, I was anxious for what was ahead.

The pre-transplant coordinator asked if I was "ready for this." I didn't know what to say. Of course I wasn't ready; is anyone ever *ready*? I was ready for something to change but was terrified by what that change would bring. On the phone, I simply responded that I was ready to head to Toronto and see what happened. Until I had to say it out loud to the coordinator on the phone, I hadn't realized that at some time during the previous month I had decided to take the gamble and try for a transplant. I had to take the risk.

Logistically, the pre-transplant coordinator said that they would like me there as soon as possible, but at least before December. Isaiah and I agreed on October as I figured that would give us enough time to sort out our lives at home in Springhill, Nova Scotia. We had to store our personal belongings somewhere, move out of our apartment, find an apartment in Toronto, and say our goodbyes to everyone in the Maritimes.

After the vacation on Prince Edward Island, I received a packet in the mail of everything I had to set up before I left the province. I had to register for medical programs, set up mail forwarding, and write up my Power of Attorney (POA). Writing the POA was something the social worker had told me to do while I was in Toronto, but I had put it off. However, now that I was in the program, I had to get to work on it.

A POA is a form that legally empowers someone else to make decisions on your behalf on the off-chance that something happens and you're unable to communicate. Medically, that means the holder of the POA gets to make the horrible decision whether or not to start life support and what kind of medical support the hospital can provide. These provisions are always better to have in writing, otherwise the next-of-kin has to blindly make decisions about care. Having your wishes written out can minimize any guilt that person might feel because they know that they are carrying out your wishes. It also protects this person legally if random family members show up demanding to have a say.

I was not concerned about Isaiah or my family not knowing what I would want, but the Toronto team still wanted something in writing. During my recreation therapy internship at a nursing home, I heard many horror stories about families brawling over end-of-life care decisions when no one knew what the person wanted and everyone thought they should have a say. Since I didn't want my family fighting in the intensive care unit (ICU)—not that I thought Amy, say, would sue Isaiah for the right to make end-of-care decisions—I figured I'd better put something on paper. I had always thought a lawyer or someone equally important had to write up the document, but apparently it was just a form in the back of Ontario's "end-of-life decision-making" booklet that needed some signatures.

During the process of writing a POA, I learned that it's important to specify what type of end-of-life care you do and do not want. It is not enough to say, "If I am not coming back to have a decent quality of life then do not prolong my death." There are many different types of "Do not Resuscitate (DNR)" and it helps to break down what type of treatment is the best decision.

Isaiah and I had the uncomfortable conversation that I didn't want to stay on a ventilator or feeding tube if I was unresponsive and wasn't going to get a transplant, or if I was post-transplant and my body was rejecting the new lungs. I also told him that if I got something acute, like chicken pox, to go ahead with treatment. I probably didn't cover everything; in fact, I'm sure I didn't, as I had no idea what type of situations to anticipate. I just didn't want to live on a ventilator for a significant period of time. I knew that I would have to be on one post-transplant, but I never wanted it to turn chronic. Thankfully, the form never had to be put to use during the transplant process, and my family didn't squabble. But it was comforting for me and Isaiah to know that if the worst happened, I would get the treatment I wanted.

During the packing process for Toronto, while trying to sort out all the logistics, I was still trying to process the move itself. I would declare at least once I day that I didn't want to move and that I was never leaving. It wasn't so much the move itself, although I do hate moving; it was more the amount of stress the moving caused and what the move represented. I had a hard time visualizing a positive outcome from the transplant. To be supportive, people would mention all the activities I could do after my surgery, but to me it was just a blank space. I was nervous to be optimistic for the future in case it all went wrong. I think my fear of the future came from growing up knowing that I would one day need a transplant when my lungs crapped out, so I had always, rightfully, equated needing a transplant with death. And that was terrifying.

Actually finding a place to live in Toronto was not an easy task. As I had only visited Toronto a handful of times, and mostly as a teenager, it was daunting to look at all the possibilities of where we could live. It wasn't an issue of there not being any places to rent, but rather that the number of choices was staggering. As someone who gets paralyzed by indecision when having to buy toilet paper, I prefer fewer options when making a decision. We knew we wanted to be downtown, and thankfully the government helped cover some of the rent as downtown Toronto prices are not exactly affordable, especially when everyone strongly suggests being as close to the hospital as possible.

Once we narrowed down our selection to a few areas of the city that were on a transit route, fit out budget, and all of our (my) demands, the decision seemed less insurmountable. We wanted a furnished place, no basements (due to the risk of mould), no mice or bedbugs (because, obviously), no carpeting or smoking, and ideally with parking. We debated whether having a car in Toronto was worth it and in the end I won out on the pro-car side. I thought it would be helpful for getting groceries or driving to the hospital on days I didn't feel well.

Once we had our short list of apartments, my cousin had the dirty job of visiting the places and weeding them out. He spent a long day looking at some superb and not-so-superb places and sent us videos and pictures. We contacted our top two choices; one of them responded that day, so we signed some forms, transferred money, and just like that, we had a place to live. It was a year lease, which seemed like a huge risk at the time because we had no idea how long we would be in Toronto. As the average wait for a transplant is eight months, plus three months "in the city" for recovery post-transplant, this meant we should expect approximately a year-long stay. However, some people get their transplant in the first three months, which would mean our stay could be as short as six months. We decided that we would take the chance. If we needed to get out of the lease early, we would cross that bridge when we came to it.

There was one final moment of panic before the move when I was called to visit the Halifax CF clinic. They didn't tell me the reason over the phone so all that came to mind was that I had cancer or that I was suddenly no longer eligible for a transplant. For some reason cancer has always been the bogeyman in my imagination, even though there are much worse issues that are more closely related to CF. I panicked the entire drive to Halifax for my appointment and during the wait. As is usually the case, it turned out my anxiety was all for naught.

I learned that my blood work showed that I was negative for antibodies for the Epstein-Barr virus (EBV, a.k.a. the mono virus). This normally wouldn't impact my life, except when it came to the lung transplant. Because the majority of the general population are positive for EBV (most people contract it when they're children and it presents as a one-day stomach bug, some people contract it as young adults and it presents as mono, and others are seemingly immune to the virus), it meant I would most likely be getting a set of lungs with the virus. Under normal circumstances, if I contracted EBV, it would be no big deal, but post-transplant, due to the massive amounts of anti-rejection medications I would be taking, I would have no immune system to fight it off.

If I got lungs with EBV, there would be a 5–10% chance that it would lead to post-transplant lymphoproliferative disorder (PTLD), which is a lymphoma-like form of cancer. Although it's treatable, it would mean lowering my anti-rejection medication, putting me at a higher risk of rejection and infection. Ideally, the doctor said, I would catch EBV before the transplant so it would not be a concern. Since I didn't particularly want to go make out with strangers, I opted to take my chances. There was also the possibility that by some fluke of genetics I might be immune to the virus. The doctor seemed much more concerned about it than I was. To me, the risk was so much lower than the risk of the actual transplant that it was way down on my list of concerns. It just added another item on my list of "cancers to watch for" post-transplant. I wish now that I had paid more attention in that meeting. I still would've had the transplant; I just may have seriously considered the idea of making out with a bunch of people.

After that appointment, and with our belongings in boxes stored with various family members, at the end of September we said goodbye to our attic apartment in Springhill and set off with our loaded-down car to the big city of Toronto.

PART II

LIFE ON THE WAIT-LIST

OCTOBER 2013 TO NOVEMBER 2014

3
TORONTO
THE WAIT IS ON

Since I grew up in a small town, I was surprised by how much I would come to enjoy living in the city. I should have expected it, because I loved living in Halifax during university, and Toronto was basically a larger, noisier Halifax with better transit. I think all my travelling to major cities helped reduce any shock I might have had about the crowds. Once you've crossed the street in Tahrir Square in Egypt or been on the Rome metro during rush hour, downtown Toronto isn't quite as intimidating. Isaiah and I drove into Toronto in our 2004 Subaru to our new apartment during the evening rush hour. The drive was chaotic, frustrating, and everything I expected from the city. After living in quiet, rural Springhill for a few years, a large city was a significant change.

Once we unloaded the car, with help from Isaiah's brother and sister-in-law, we settled into our new tiny, furnished apartment. While the apartment itself was a standard one-bedroom space, the amenities in the building were marvellous. There was a pool, a gym, a hot tub, a terrace, and barbeques to use any time. The small outdoor space was often an escape for me on days when I didn't want to go anywhere but still felt as though I needed a change of scenery and some fresh air—although on hot days, the filtered apartment air sometimes felt better than the outside city air. We had no problem adapting to city life by jaywalking with the crowd, shoving our way on to busy streetcars, and becoming experts in aggressive city driving. I loved it.

On October 8, 2013, we had the big listing meeting with the transplant coordinator and the transplant surgeon. The transplant coordinator reviewed everything in the Almighty Transplant Manual, my POA form, what to do when I got The Call, and how to stay healthy while waiting for The Call—a.k.a., "don't touch anything or socialize with anyone." It was all straightforward.

We were informed of a support group at the hospital that met every Wednesday at noon for people on the lung transplant list as well as their caregivers. Although some weeks were open sessions, most of the time they brought in different professionals to talk about various topics such as depression, physiotherapy regimes, or what to expect post-transplant. The support group sounded great, except for the fact that I wasn't allowed to attend. Because the current infection control requirement was for people with CF to stay at least two metres apart at all times, no one with CF was allowed to attend the support meetings for fear we would swap potentially deadly germs. Our caregivers, however, could attend and relay information to us if there was a topic we were interested in.

The paranoia about keeping people with CF away from each other is relatively new when it comes to infection control. When Amy and I were younger, we attended a weekend family camp organized by the Riverview Kinettes where we tie-dyed T-shirts, ran around wildly, and watched movies with other children who had CF. It was refreshing to be around new people without having to explain why we needed aerosol masks or physiotherapy like we had to do at every other summer camp we attended. We also had Christmas parties with the Moncton chapter of CF Canada, where the families would get together to share a meal, exchange presents, and talk. I don't remember bonding with any of the other children with CF but that's more because I'm introverted than because we didn't have the opportunity. The camps and Christmas parties were all stopped once CF Canada introduced policies to keep people with CF away from each other. Now the only time to see other people with CF is during the annual Walk to Make Cystic Fibrosis History, and even then, those of us with CF wear green bandanas so we can identify one another from afar and keep our distance. Social media has made it possible for people to connect without having to meet in person, which I think has been a huge advantage to the CF community.

Even if I had been allowed, I'm not sure I would have attended the support group at the hospital, but I think it would've been beneficial to have something for the people with CF. My outlet for stress was writing posts for the blog I started at the outset of the transplant process. The blog helped in keeping my friends and family updated on my life as well as giving me a place to channel my emotions during the various stages of transplant. Isaiah tends to not get bothered by much, so he didn't feel as though the support group would benefit him. And when he is stressed, he doesn't want to talk about his feelings to a large group of strangers. He attended one meeting the entire time I was listed and that was because while I was at physiotherapy one day, the physiotherapist told him that she was talking, that he needed to go, and stared him down until he agreed to attend. She then walked with him to the meeting. There was no getting out of it that day. He said it was pretty boring.

The surgeon meeting the day of listing was informative and more overwhelming than the one with the transplant coordinator. Both Isaiah and I had to sign several papers stating that we understood the risks of the operation. The surgeon listed all the possible complications: infection, cardiac arrest, stroke, pneumonia, death, etc. He said that for people with CF, the rate of death during the surgery is two to three out of one hundred patients, but he would put my odds at, "less than 1%" if the surgery happened immediately because I was young and relatively healthy—"healthy" being a subjective term.

Although I had prepared myself to hear the play-by-play on how the surgery would proceed, he didn't get into the details, which was fine by me. I had read an overview; that was enough. He did feel obliged to mention that I couldn't have a boob job or any cosmetic surgery done on my chest post-transplant. Also, they wouldn't do any cosmetic adaptations during the actual surgery. I hadn't brought this up as a possibility so I'm not sure why he felt he needed to clarify that for me. Do people actually ask to have other procedures done since the doctor "is there" anyway? Wouldn't you want them to focus more on important tasks like transplanting the lungs or making sure your heart is still pumping? Not for the first time in my life, I thought how people are weird.

At the end of the day, my coordinator filed all my paperwork, and I was officially listed for a double-lung transplant. The wait was on.

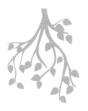

4

PRE-TRANSPLANT PHYSIOTHERAPY

STAYING STRONG

The Toronto lung transplant program accepts people for transplants earlier health-wise than other programs across Canada because they want everyone on a regular exercise routine before the transplant. They've found that people who exercise regularly tend to be less symptomatic while waiting and have a better chance at recovery, as their bodies are stronger to undergo and recover from surgery. Therefore, physiotherapy is an important part of the pre-transplant process. The physio room at the TGH is set up similar to a standard gym, only the weights are lighter, the equipment can be modified, and instead of personal trainers, there are physiotherapists monitoring everyone. Everyone in the lung transplant program at the TGH—roughly between sixty and eighty people at any time—is required to attend a physiotherapy program three times a week. Most people on the transplant list end up doing their physiotherapy at the TGH. Those living outside the city usually attend a place closer to home twice a week and commute in weekly so the Toronto team can continue to follow them.

The physiotherapists at TGH were exceptional and would closely monitor everyone's progress through progress cards (yellow for pre-transplant, green for post-transplant, and blue for "out of town"). They wrote down what they expected to be done and then I would write down what I actually did that day. I also recorded my heart rate and oxygen levels, both before and after cardio and weights. After the initial introduction day, everyone was more or less left alone to do their own thing. The exercise routine was basically the same for every person: approximately a half hour of cardio, then some weights and stretches. I did fifteen minutes on the stationary bike and twenty minutes on the treadmill. Those who could not use the treadmills used the stationary arm or leg machines while sitting in a chair. The physiotherapists would try to check in at least once a week to see how I was progressing or feeling. They would answer any questions, fix any problems, and make changes accordingly. After each physio session, the physiotherapists would review and sign the cards, sometimes making notes or comments such as, "Perhaps you need to increase your weights," or, "I think you should walk at a higher speed."

After the first week or so, I fell into a routine and soon got bored. I was not used to going to a gym and having to exercise regularly. I wanted to switch things up and do something more exciting. I had always been a fairly active person as much as my energy level would allow. As children, our parents encouraged me and my siblings to be as active as possible, taking us on long hikes and bike rides in the summer and cross-country skiing and skating in the winter. They are both active people, so it was natural that they would pass that on to their children. Besides that, it was also important to stay as active as possible for my and Amy's lung health. David was the only child who got Dad's love of playing team sports. I played soccer in grade six and was quite terrible. That was enough of team sports for me.

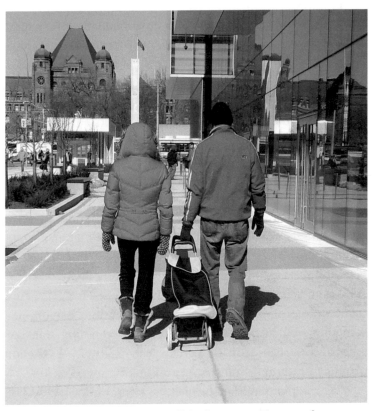

Allison and her partner, Isaiah, walk in downtown Toronto after a physio session at the Toronto General Hospital in March 2014. Isaiah is pulling a cart containing Allison's oxygen canister. (Sarah Jacques)

I had also stayed active through horseback riding. It started with Amy wanting a horse, so Mom and Dad bought a "family horse" when we were in middle school. Dad says it was one of the few concessions they made for us because we had CF. In retrospect, Mom feels that maybe they shouldn't have, based on all the current research that shows an increased health risk from bacteria that grows in mouldy hay and barns. But we didn't know any of that at the time, so Amy and I took riding lessons and loved it. We were hooked. Sharing a horse isn't exactly practical in the long run, so I used money I won from a "Tell Us About Your Accomplishments" hospital contest and bought myself a horse. (I wrote about how I took sewing lessons and made myself a quilt with much help from Mom.) I used money from our family paper route to pay for board and all the other costs that come with owning a horse. David eventually joined us in our love of riding, bought his own horse, and we all spent a lot of time riding through the nearby woods and fields. Amy stopped riding regularly when the family horse had to be put down, but she still joined David and me occasionally.

When my first horse had to be put down because her back legs kept giving out, I wondered how I could afford to get a second one. That is when I looked to the Children's Wish Foundation. Amy and I had always been told that the Wish Foundation and other similar programs were to be used for "kids who were actually sick" and not for us. I'm pretty sure this attitude has impacted how I feel about my disability: it's something you manage and move on, not something that warrants special treatment. However, I badly wanted a horse and couldn't afford one on my own. So I applied and told my parents afterwards that I had filled out the application. And I was approved! (To this day, Amy remains slightly bitter that she never got a Wish.) After a long search that took Mom and me all over the Maritimes so I could try out different horses, I found

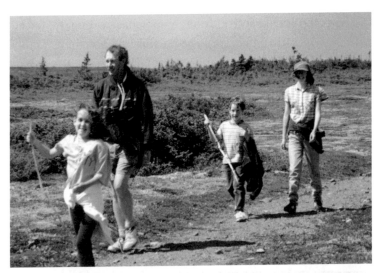

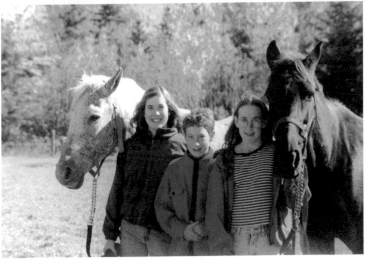

TOP: Allison (left) hiking in Labrador in 1996 with her father, David, brother, David, and sister, Amy. Travelling and hiking were pursuits that the family enjoyed together. Allison was instilled with a love of both that continues to this day. (Donna Watson) BOTTOM: Allison (right) and her siblings were encouraged to stay active through horseback riding. The family friend's farm where the horses were stabled was like a second home to Allison. (Dianne Bannister)

the perfect one, a beautiful sorrel quarter horse named Sydney. Riding horses kept me healthy and active in a way that no other sport did.

Because none of the regular exercise I was accustomed to involved a gym or treadmill, it took some adjusting to the formal routine of the physiotherapy room. Eventually though, while I was still bored, I had the routine down; I felt as though I could do it in my sleep. The repetition meant that I didn't have to think about what I was doing or stress about a new program. I arrived, did my thing, and left.

Isaiah often attended with me to help keep track of my numbers, fetch me water, and clean the machines and weights for me after I had used them. It was fairly boring for him because the physiotherapists don't want the support people exercising alongside the transplant people. In fact, I heard them tell several support people to stop lifting weights and take a seat. It's probably a liability thing even though the support people were simply trying to motivate their loved ones. Isaiah usually just sat in a chair and read, unless he got sucked into a conversation with another bored support person. He accompanied me more and more often as the year progressed and my health declined because it became harder for me to find the energy to both do the exercises and wipe everything down afterward.

Everyone at the "gym" was waiting for a lung transplant like me, so this was pretty much the only time I saw people who were also listed. It turned into a social event, although I never met anyone else waiting who also had CF because the scheduling intentionally separated us. I was fine with that, because Amy and I tended to stick together and never sought out other people with CF. After the camps and social events we attended as kids were closed down, I didn't try to find a community online until after I had my transplant. The CF groups are usually fine, but it seems it doesn't take long before they're taken over by people who just want to talk about religion or the power of the latest trendy cure. (Inhaling silver, anyone? Only fifty dollars a bottle if you buy it from me!) We've found a few more people now, thanks to my experience of having had a transplant, but overall we still tend to stick to ourselves. I'm not sure if it's an emotional survival mechanism (the more people you know with CF, the greater the odds are of watching them die) or if we're just antisocial that way.

The people I met at physiotherapy were all older than me and most of them had pulmonary fibrosis, COPD, or occasionally a type of lung cancer. Despite my introversion, over the year of waiting, I got to know people and would see others be listed, transplanted, and discharged three months post-transplant, while I continued to wait. It was hard not to get bitter at times when I saw people come in and leave before me; at the same time, many of those people were much sicker than I was, so I knew they were higher priority.

One of the big misconceptions about transplants is that it's a "first come, first served" system. People would often ask me where I was on the transplant list. I had to inform them that it didn't work that way. The only real differentiation between people was whether or not they were in "group one" or "group two"—basically low or high priority. After that, the decision is based on blood type, infections, lung size, and how close the person is to dying. If there were two exact matches on the waiting list, the team would then go with who had been waiting the longest, but that would be toward the end of their consideration priorities.

⸙

The first week at physiotherapy, I had to do a six-minute walk test, which was then repeated about every three months. A six-minute walk test consists of walking up and down a hallway as fast as possible for six minutes. The goal is to do as many laps as possible. There is no real data for an "average walk test" from the "average person," which I find bizarre. Much like pulmonary function tests, it's more of a comparison to your last number as a way of indicating if your body is getting stronger or weaker.

The first walk test I did was in Halifax during my pre-assessment workup, so the team wanted me to repeat it because it had been over six months. At that point I was still only using oxygen "upon exertion" so they lent me a little oxygen cart to haul an oxygen canister up and down the hallway for the walk. I managed to trip over it, run it over the physiotherapist's foot, and drop it on the ground. I'm super-coordinated that way. The actual number showed no real change since my last test, which was a pleasant surprise, showing that my endurance hadn't declined over those six months.

The worst part about physiotherapy for me was the self-reflection. I've never been good with self-reflection and they used the Borg Scale, which is all about rating how the body feels on a scale of one to ten before and after exertion. I never knew how to answer the subjective questions such as, "How tired are your legs on a scale from one to ten?" and, "How bad is your breathing on a scale of one to ten?" If ten is the worst I can imagine, then probably a two...or three...maybe? They wanted me to be exercising at an exertion of "three to four," which is described as "mild to moderate breathing," but I never knew what that meant because people would often tell me that I seemed short of breath when I felt fine. As the weeks went on, I settled into a habit of saying three if the workout felt easy, four if I was breathing heavily, and five if I frequently coughed. I just made up numbers when they asked about my legs since I usually went from "not noticing my legs" to "my legs are numb" after a walk test. I'm not sure how that translated on a one-to-ten scale. I assumed if my legs gave out, that would be a ten.

The scale stressed me out because I wanted to be the perfect patient and give the right answer. I'm not good with subjective questions and I wanted something on which to measure the numbers. I felt as if I was making stuff up, I was giving a wrong answer. Of course, there were no wrong answers and it was more about how I felt compared to the day before, but even that was hard. I preferred to base my health and feeling from my oxygen levels and heart rate numbers, tangible numbers. If something went up or down with those, to my thinking, that was a better indication of how hard the workout was.

As the months progressed, I found that I got stronger on the treadmill and reached a plateau with my weights. It took a long time to build up to ten-pound weights (the max they had in the room) because the physiotherapists only wanted people to increase their weights one pound at a time. Regular exercise increased my appetite, and as a result, I managed to gain some much-needed weight during the year. I know most people exercise to lose weight, but for me exercising is an appetite stimulant and has always helped me gain weight. I reached a weight plateau eventually, but exercising did more for my hunger than my other plan, which was to watch cooking shows. (Exercising while watching cooking shows would almost be the perfect appetite stimulant.)

I tried not to miss too many physiotherapy appointments, even though it was tempting to stay in bed most mornings. The one thing that made me go on the mornings when it was -20° c with wind-chill or when I hadn't slept well the previous night, was that if I didn't go I had to call the physiotherapists to cancel. This was fine if no one was there and I got the voicemail, but I found one of the physiotherapists kind of intimidating and being grilled by her on why I wasn't showing up was not how I wanted to start my day. If I was feeling legitimately terrible, Isaiah would call while I slept, but he refused to do so if I was just being lazy. So, off I went.

Three months into the waiting stage, I had my second six-minute walk test, which was about on par with my first. I always stressed over the walk tests as they drained all my energy, and I wanted to do better than the one before. Although the walk tests were taxing, attending physiotherapy was great for my overall health. The regular exercise, as well as the effort it took just getting to the hospital three times a week, helped keep my body functioning fairly well, even as my lungs declined.

Once my lung function started dropping, physiotherapy became more and more of a chore and my last two walk tests pre-transplant were absolutely miserable. I didn't have enough energy to care about my last one, which ended up being a good thing because I hadn't realized how much the walk test influenced whether or not I got bumped up to status two, or "high priority." At the time, my CF doctors at St. Mike's were trying to get me levelled up, but as I kept pushing myself at physiotherapy and collapsing at home afterward, the physiotherapists didn't notice my declining health as quickly.

It wasn't until I did so poorly on my last walk test and was coughing more frequently (it's unbelievable that was even possible) while exercising that they finally noted I wasn't doing so well. I think it took throwing up in the room to get them to notice. While I wasn't the first person to throw up in the treadmill room, it was still embarrassing when it happened. Isaiah grabbed a garbage can for me and I tried to minimize it as much as possible, but instead I puked up my guts and continued to dry heave for a while. The physiotherapists have seen it all and were not fazed. They told me to go home and not return until I had seen a doctor. It turned out to be one of my last pre-transplant physio days. I was hospitalized at St. Mike's soon after.

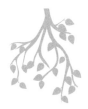

5

TUBING STRAPPED
TO MY FACE

little more than a week into life in Toronto, a representative from the oxygen supply company arrived at
our new apartment to make sure everything had been
set up properly for me. I had brought some compressed oxygen
tanks with me, as well as my big oxygen compressor, but the
Toronto team thought it would be best if I switched to the liquid oxygen tanks. These would be easier than the compressed
air because I could refill them at the hospital. The company provided me with a small, portable liquid oxygen tank, about the
size of a four-slice toaster, weighing around 4.5 kilograms when
full. They also provided me with a large tank so I could fill the

smaller one at home. The large tank looked like an oversized R2-D2, and thankfully it was on wheels because it was heavy and not easily portable. The company sent someone with their oxygen truck to fill it every other week.

The day the representative arrived for consultation, I was not yet using oxygen full-time, even though the physiotherapists had strongly suggested I should. I was still in denial that this was something I needed when I wasn't exercising. While the man was waiting for the paperwork from his office to get sorted out, he took my vitals with and without oxygen, both resting and walking. For context, a normal oxygen saturation rate is between 95 and 100%. While sitting, I was 98% on oxygen and 94% on room air, which was excellent; however, after five minutes of strolling down the hallway on room air, I had dropped below 88%.

While it's true that people had mentioned I should use oxygen even while casually walking, no one had shown me the data of what was happening in my body. For most people, if their oxygen drops below 90%, they will feel short of breath. For me, it felt no different than when I was at 95%. I mean, I noticed when I walked up a hill or a flight of stairs and got a bit of a headache, but it was never something I noticed while strolling around. Seeing the numbers helped knock it into my brain that I truly did need to wear oxygen while doing everyday activities. Just because I had no symptoms that indicated my oxygen levels were dropping didn't meant that the rest of my body was fine—a low oxygen saturation meant that my heart and body worked harder to get enough oxygen. No wonder I was tired all the time. (Low oxygen can also cause swelling in the feet as well as skin discolouration, which never happened to me.)

The oxygen supply man left me with these comforting words: "Most people with CF only get their transplant after a flare-up, when they're incredibly close to death." I responded that sounded terrible because it meant people would be less healthy for the recovery process and I would like to not go that route. He concluded by advising me that getting sick would be the best way to get the transplant, so if I got a cold I should complain a lot and let everyone know, and then I could be bumped up to the "high priority" group. I laughed him off, saying he was cynical, without knowing how prophetic his words would turn out to be.

I started wearing oxygen while walking around the city, which I grudgingly admitted helped with my energy levels. I still hated wearing it around the apartment, but I soon found myself putting it on more and more. I eventually bought myself an oxygen saturation monitor, which helped me know when my levels were dropping so I would be able to see, outside of physiotherapy, when I had to strap on the oxygen and when I was okay without it. I still resisted having to wear oxygen on a daily basis. I hated feeling like a sick person, and having to haul around oxygen administered through a tube on my face was a constant reminder that I was sick. I knew rationally that I was ill—otherwise I wouldn't be in Toronto waiting for a transplant—but since my health was relatively stable, I didn't have a constant reminder. Wearing oxygen was suddenly that constant reminder that made people feel comfortable approaching me to ask what was wrong.

I was accustomed to explaining CF to random people. I had to explain it often on my and David's cross-Canada cycling trip in 2008. We decided to cycle across the country on a bit of a whim. David mentioned on Thanksgiving about going with one of his friends; I invited myself along and started planning. I mapped out a route across the country based on 80- to 100-kilometre distances and made packing lists for each of us. When the friend backed out, we decided if we were going, it should be an awareness campaign for CF. The people of Kin Canada and our then-hometown of Petitcodiac, New Brunswick, were intensely supportive of our trip and organized host families on our route who gave us shelter and meals; some even arranged social events. We also stayed with friends and family and tented on the nights when we didn't know anyone in the area. The logistics of a trip that length while having CF meant I carried my medication as well as a battery-operated aerosol machine that was necessary when we camped off-road. We didn't have the space in our bike panniers for a hundred-day supply of medication so I mailed myself care packages to people who agreed to host us in strategic locations across the country.

Each region of the country had its own charm. We visited parts of Canada that we otherwise would have never seen and met many wonderful people. People took us in on our trip with no background knowledge of who we were, fed us burgers and beer in hotel parking lots, and didn't hesitate to drive along the highway looking for my sleeping bag upon discovering that it had fallen off my bike. We heard the same jokes, "You know what they say about the weather in *name of region/province*. If you don't like it, just wait five minutes!" and watched the hockey playoffs in many homes that cheered for different teams.

The trip was a "figure it out on the go" adventure with a steep learning curve. David and I were determined we would complete the trip, taking each day as it arrived. We motivated each other when it was a struggle to keep going and took care of each other if we had an off day. I'll admit, this more often fell on David to make sure the camp was okay and to do dishes while I went to sleep at 7:00 P.M. We were able to pass the time discussing nonsense, singing stupid songs, and generally finding humour in most situations—a family trait that continues to carry us through life.

There are major and minor life lessons that I learned from the trip. Major lessons included accepting help from people, although I continue to work on that, travelling minimally, and it's okay to not meet your daily goal if it means learning that you'll be better off for the next day. Minor lessons included learning that crows will eat food if it's not packed away properly, a pack of bacon will immediately burn in a tiny frying pan when cooked on a camping stove, and 8 kmh is the speed at which Northern Ontario mosquitoes give up their relentless attack.

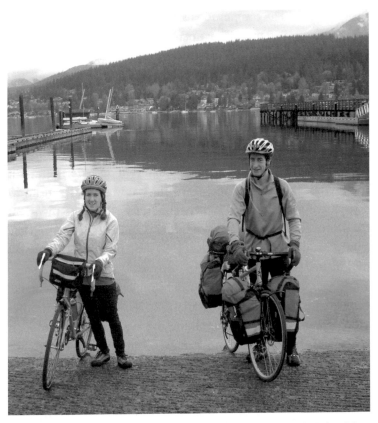

Allison and her brother, David, near Port Coquitlam, British Columbia, at the start of their ninety-one–day cross-Canada cycling trip in 2008. (Gord Stone)

Ninety-one days after we started, we pedalled into St. John's on August 1. Incredibly, it felt as though we had simply completed another day and not that we had just biked for more than seven thousand kilometres. It feels more significant now whenever I'm on a road trip and think, *I cycled all of this* or, *Wow, this highway is endless, I can't believe I pedalled through here.*

There are many things I would change about the trip if we had a do-over but all of them are logistical details like packing differently and eating at more restaurants. I wouldn't change the trip itself. The passing of time has smoothed out my memories of that summer to the fun and exhausting three months I spent with my brother.

People we stayed with during our cycling trip usually knew CF as a "children's lung disease," but not much beyond that. There were always some questions and explanations needed when I took a handful of pills before a meal, started an aerosol mask in the wee hours of the morning, or when David started beating on my back. Aerosol masks and chest percussions were the main treatment for the faulty lung component of CF. Every person has a different combination of the number and frequency of aerosol masks they take, but generally, it's one or two masks twice a day. The frequency and number of masks increases as a person's lung health declines. While it's not a common treatment anymore, when Amy and I were born, the best practice was to do chest percussions post-aerosol mask by literally beating around the area to help loosen any mucus in the lungs. The idea behind the chest percussions was that after an aerosol mask, the thick mucus in the lungs would be looser so it could be beaten out of the body. The new generation of kids with CF use hand-held breathing exercise machines or a vibrating vest that are supposed to work as well, or better, than the old-fashioned chest percussions. I've tried a few of them but up until my transplant, I was still doing the chest percussions because I found them the most effective.

Amy and I called the practice "physio" and had it done every morning and evening with five minutes of percussion per lung lobe. While it looked like it might hurt, it felt good. The percussions only hurt if the person was doing it with a flat hand (instead of cupping the hands) or if they were wearing heavy jewellery and beating you with their rings. I always felt better and could breathe easier afterward. If I was lazy or slept in and skipped physio, I would notice during the day, so it was rare that I missed out.

When Amy and I were travelling, we would often get a lot of questions about what we were doing if we had a shared room at a hostel or had to do our physio on an overnight train. For whatever reason, everyone seemed to understand if we said it was a medical issue related to asthma. *Asthma* clearly translates more easily into other languages than CF and is much more common, so people understood if we started with that. It wasn't exactly the truth, but as we were never going to see these people again, it didn't matter what we told them as long as they understood that it was a medical matter.

Whenever I went anywhere new by myself for an extended period of time, I would have to get someone to do my physio for me. As a child, summer camp was the only time when it was an issue for me, but then my parents arranged to have it done with the student nurse. Every morning I would go to the nurse's cabin to do my aerosol masks and physiotherapy. I don't remember feeling like I was being singled out, but I did hate having to get up earlier than everyone else and missing some evening activities. I don't think I talked about it with the other kids unless they asked; after all, what twelve-year-old wants to be the different one who needs extra treatment?

My first year of university, my parents set up physiotherapy with the resident assistant on my floor of the dormitory. It didn't take me long to ask my new friends to do it instead. It's a bit of an awkward conversation to have with someone new: "Hi! I'm Allison, can you please beat on my back for five minutes?" But it does help build a friendship.

By the time I spent a summer at a horse camp in Ireland as a camp counsellor when I was nineteen, I was much better at harassing strangers to pound on my back. I was there for the entire summer while the other counsellors stayed for two weeks to a month. It was tiresome to teach the new staff person every time they rotated through, so I probably didn't get it done as much as I should've. I say "camp counsellor" because that's what I put on my resumé, but in fact it was just me and one other (rotating) person in charge of twenty kids from around Europe. The kids would ride horses and learn English; our job was to provide evening entertainment, which usually meant playing soccer in the fields.

Eventually, I became accustomed to wearing oxygen in public. It wasn't until February 2014, when I got a head cold, that I started wearing it while sleeping. I hadn't been acutely sick until that point, but I knew it was just a matter of time before I caught something during that cold Toronto winter. While I was sick, I felt much better wearing the oxygen and seemed to sleep better. Once I got over the cold, I continued wearing it at night because by then I had adjusted to sleeping with the nasal prongs. I figured by that point, my oxygen levels were probably dropping below reasonable levels while I slept.

The only problem I had sleeping with oxygen was that, occasionally, I would roll around during my sleep and wake up wrapped up in the tubing. I had a slight fear of strangling myself with the tubing during the night. While death by oxygen tubing would be an ironic way to die, it was not the way I wanted to go out. After February, I wore oxygen pretty much 24/7. I took a few hours off now and then to give my nose a break from the dry air and to rest my oxygen compressor, but those breaks got further and further apart.

While outside of the apartment, I usually carried my oxygen tank around in a small cart that I could pull behind me. The first one was destroyed after a few months because the wheels couldn't handle the abuse of being bumped over curbs all the time. Cart 2.0 was a bit fancier, put on many more kilometres, and was still going strong when we left. However, if I was going somewhere with limited space, like a concert or crowded museum, I would opt to put the tank in my backpack instead. It was a good system.

Eventually, I didn't notice that I was wearing oxygen. It just became another thing I had to deal with, like taking medication or doing aerosol masks. Gradually, I stopped being self-conscious about wearing oxygen in public and realized that few people in Toronto cared. Some people would offer me a seat on the bus if it was crowded, which I appreciated and usually declined unless it had been a long day. I wasn't used to wearing a sign of my disability. I wasn't accustomed to the sly, questioning looks on the subway. I was fine explaining CF and lung failure, but it had usually been done on my own terms. There is a difference between deciding to disclose your disability to someone and having it shouted out for you.

6

THE WINTER OF
MY WAITING

While downtown Toronto would not initially be my first choice of a place to wait for a lung transplant due to the smog, traffic, and number of people, it ended up being terrific because there was so much to do to distract myself when I wasn't at physiotherapy or other appointments. I tried my best to approach living in Toronto as a one-time experience that I should take advantage of to the best of my abilities. Isaiah and I tried to be tourists, trying to see as much of the city as possible. Touring Toronto is easy to do if one has unlimited funds, which was, unfortunately, not our case. But we did find options for those of us with budgets if we looked and planned carefully.

We planned for all the free or cheap nights for the museums and shows. The best program we found was through the city library, where we took full advantage of their Museum and Arts Pass (MAP) program. With our library cards, which we acquired as soon as we arrived, we got free passes for the city's more "educational" museums. Using the passes, we visited every major museum and the zoo as often as we could. The passes were great for me: because we didn't have to pay entrance fees, I didn't feel pressured to see the entire place in one visit. Not that I was ever externally pressured by Isaiah: "If we pay, we're going to see the entire thing!" It was more of a self-determination thing, that if I paid for the visit, I wanted to get my money's worth. With the passes I didn't feel bad if we went to the zoo and only saw a few of the animals.

We were gifted an annual pass for the Royal Ontario Museum (ROM), which is a first-rate museum that held excellent visiting exhibitions during our time there. Our pass also allowed us to take visitors, so whenever anyone visited, off we went to the ROM. We were also generously gifted a season's pass to the theatre, which was fantastic and kept us busy. We attended many shows that winter. While some were better than others, they were all brilliant. We visited various markets, street festivals, and whatever else was happening for free around the city.

While part of the motivation for exploring the city was to see the place we now called home, another major part was to keep my anxiety at bay. During the lead-up to moving to Toronto, while I would have moments of anxiety or panic, if asked, I wouldn't have said that I was generally anxious. However, after being listed, *anxious* would have been the top word I would've used to describe myself. I was beyond paranoid about missing The Call.

The first few nights I was listed, I woke up panicked every few hours that I had missed The Call and had to check my phone before I could get back to sleep. Every time the phone rang with an unlisted or unknown number, I would get an adrenaline rush in case it was The Call. The adrenaline and panic never completely stopped but they did tone down as the months dragged on. Getting the "you've won a cruise!" calls were annoying but the worst were when there was a person on the other end of a blocked number (calls from the hospital always came up on the caller ID as "blocked"). If they didn't introduce themselves right way, I would start having a mild panic attack.

"Hello?"

"Hello, is this Allison?"

"Yes..."

"Hi Allison, how are you doing today?"

"Fine! What do you want? Are you giving me new lungs?"

They were always calling about something useless like a new credit card or bank loan offer. The entire interaction never stopped being frustrating. If I missed a call and there was no message, I would also irrationally think that I had missed The Call, even though the hospital reassured me that they would leave a message and call back ten minutes later and would also call my pager and Isaiah's phone. My rational side knew it was a telemarketer, but I was only ever reassured after I googled the number.

I also panicked a bit every time my phone battery was running low, fearful of the chance that the battery would run out and the hospital wouldn't be able to get a hold of me. This also wasn't rational—anxiety rarely is. I found it was hard to focus at a concert or show because part of me was always concentrating on the purse in my hand, waiting for the pager (set to vibrate) to go off. I spent the first few minutes in a new place or situation visualizing what would happen if I got The Call. Because of the anxiety, I had a hard time sleeping. My brain was a constant whirlwind of *What would happen if...?* so I continued to listen to podcasts to lull me to sleep.

When I finally made it to sleep, it didn't always help because I had vivid dreams for the first few months about missing The Call. Eventually those stopped but were soon replaced by ones where I was hanging out with my family somewhere in the Maritimes when I would suddenly realize that I needed to be in Ontario for my transplant. I don't know if my subconscious was working through missing my family and the Maritimes or if it was a new way to wake me up panicked in the middle of the night, but either way, it worked. Thanks, subconscious!

I know it sounds as though going out to activities or events enhanced my anxiety, and while it may have slightly, it did help to take my mind off the situation for a while. After all the hospital visits and physiotherapy, I needed nights where I dressed in something more exciting than exercise clothes and spent an evening around non-hospital people.

Realistically, I didn't expect to get The Call during the first three months. If I had, I'm not positive I would've gone through with the transplant. During that time, I settled into a routine, and booking shows for the future gave me activities to look forward to so I wouldn't get discouraged about the wait. There was, of course, always a risk in booking plans in advance in case I got The Call and couldn't attend, but the reward of having something to look forward to outweighed the risk of losing some money.

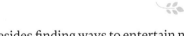

Besides finding ways to entertain myself in Toronto, I found that I felt better when I did crafty things at home. I struggled with this when I was first put off work, not knowing what I was going to do with myself all day. Unsurprisingly, I found it easy to fill my days. As I couldn't do as many of the physical activities I enjoyed, I had to learn some new activities. I learned how to knit and returned to my childhood love of painting and drawing. I found projects to try from Pinterest, some more successful than others.

And then, in February 2014, I found pottery. As part of the MAP passes, we went to the Gardiner, the ceramics museum, and while we were looking at the pottery, I noticed that they offered both drop-in classes and eight-week courses. I thought it sounded fun and tried to convince Isaiah to attend with me. As pottery is not even close to being an interest of his, I waited until Amy came to visit before attending a drop-in class. Sometimes drop-in classes are only for those "in the loop," so I was nervous going by myself even though the sign said beginners were welcome. Amy and I went and had a ball. We used a pottery wheel and made a giant mess but somehow managed to produce two wobbly bowls by the end of the two hours. I returned with Mom in two weeks when the bowls were ready and we glazed away. In the end, our bowls were kind of a mess but in a beautiful way. I loved being able to get my hands dirty as well as using my creative side when it came to glazing and etching the clay.

Pottery arrived in my life at the right time, because February was a hard month for me health-wise. I had a bit of a head cold in January and although it didn't seem to move to my lungs, it still knocked me down. My lung function dropped, and while I wasn't at the point of feeling exhausted from waiting, the cold Toronto winter was a struggle. Toronto is not a pleasant place in the winter, and the winter of my waiting happened to be the coldest in ten years or something like that. The bitter wind never stopped howling through the wind tunnels between the buildings. My shoulders and back were knotted with tension as my body froze up every time I went outside. It would feel as if my lungs were seizing, and I usually ended up having a coughing fit shortly after leaving a building. I ended up driving more around the city because I couldn't stand the cold while waiting for the bus.

There were a few days that winter when I wanted the transplant to happen so I wouldn't have to deal with going outside into the cold to get to physiotherapy. These were also the first inklings I had of not knowing why I was putting myself through the struggle of waiting for a transplant and thinking how much I just wanted the wait to end. I wasn't feeling lonely, because there had been no shortage of family around; I was simply worn down.

So with much encouragement from my family, I signed up for the spring session of pottery tableware–making. I was hesitant about it at first. I wasn't sure I should commit to an eight-week program, but signing up proved to be good for my soul (or optimism, or good spirits, or whatever you want to call it). It gave me something to look forward to, and similar to the art classes I had taken in December, having a scheduled activity made it so that if I didn't get the transplant over the eight-week program, it would be okay because then I wouldn't have to worry about making up the classes. The first class had a steep learning curve, but everyone was extremely friendly and walked me through what to do. I spent afternoons before and after classes sketching out ideas and searching Etsy for unrealistic ideas of ceramics I could make.

Instead of lying awake at night wondering what would happen if I did get The Call, I would dream up what to make at pottery class. It was also terrific to meet people outside of hospital-land who I could converse with about normal-people problems like mothers-in-law with dementia, co-workers, and horrible pets. It was relaxing and got me out of the apartment once a week to somewhere other than the hospital. I did two eight-week sessions before my transplant and it helped pass the time. When I wasn't in sessions, I attended the drop-in classes. I started taking my visitors to the drop-in classes, which became one of my key getaway spots from stress. There was something about getting my hands dirty and being creative that was incredibly therapeutic.

All in all, Isaiah and I found many ways to entertain ourselves in Toronto. He had weekly board games nights, sometimes twice a week, to get him out of the house and have a break from me and the hospital. It was unfortunate that both of our activities outside the apartment coincided on Wednesday nights because this meant we only had one night a week apart. Despite that, we somehow managed not to kill each other after spending almost two years together in our one-bedroom apartment. It also helped that we had some family in the area, so we could visit their homes for yummy meals, dips in a pool, and board games nights. We both enjoyed living in Toronto, mostly, I think, because we knew we wouldn't be staying forever.

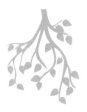

7

THE DECLINE

JUNE 2014 TO
SEPTEMBER 2014

My other regularly scheduled events during my waiting time, besides physiotherapy, were clinic visits, both at the TGH and St. Mike's. The St. Mike's team looked at everything regarding the CF part of my life and the TGH team looked at everything else regarding the transplant. Even though there was overlap between those two general aspects, I was shocked by the lack of communication between the hospitals. The staff kept reassuring me that they talked to each other, but the fact that they never seemed to know which tests I had just done at one hospital or the other made me skeptical about how well they were communicating.

Before the transplant, most of my clinic visits were at St. Mike's. The team there was in charge of keeping my lungs as stable as possible, making medication changes, and deciding if I needed hospitalization. When I first moved to Toronto, I saw them roughly once a month. By the summer, when my lung function was starting to drop, I was seeing them every other week, sometimes weekly.

The clinic appointments with the TGH team were every month, or every two months, depending on which doctor was booking the appointments. Those clinics seemed to involve a lot of waiting and then a ten-second doctor's appointment in which I would share the results of my latest lung function test, the doctor would ask what I had been doing at St. Mike's, if I had any other test results, and send me on my way. While it seemed like a giant waste of time and energy for both of us, it was comforting to know there were so many teams looking out for me so I would be less likely to slip through the cracks.

I managed to stay relatively stable from October 2013 until June 2014. Then my lung function started to drop. That's when I started seeing the staff at St. Mike's more often than I wanted. My lung function hit a new low with a FEV1 of 0.77, which was about 21% of my expected output. The doctor at St. Mike's suspected it was due to inflammation and not an infection since I didn't have any cold symptoms. (Just to refresh, an infection is when the body comes in contact with an infectious organism, i.e., bacteria, fungi, or a virus, whereas inflammation is a reaction of the body to a stimulus or injury, i.e., allergies to pollen, asthma flare-up to cold weather, or localized swelling after a bear mauling. An infection can cause inflammation but inflammation is not necessarily caused by infection.)

My oxygen saturation levels also dropped a bit in June, and I had a cold that knocked my energy down significantly more than it should have. I was given a new puffer for the inflammation, which jumped my lung function back up to 28% after a few weeks. I had energy to burn and could walk around the city much longer than before. I didn't crash out as much after physiotherapy and was able to stay up longer at night. It was a marvellous high that I hoped would never end. Unfortunately, it came crashing down at the end of July. I was given oral antibiotics, which helped until I crashed out again in August. They tried me on a variety of oral antibiotic cocktails but nothing seemed to work for longer than a week or two.

Then in September, I got a whopper of a head cold. I realized then, while lying in bed, how little it took to knock my energy levels down to scary lows. When I was feeling "fine," I never dwelled on how chronically sick I was or the reduced reserve my body had left. Before this, I had always been able to keep going and push through a cold or infection, but that ability completely disappeared. It scared me to not have any energy because of a head cold and it was a stark reminder of how limited my lungs and body had become.

The day in September I was hit with the head cold and I wasn't able to get out of bed, I called the CF clinic to set up a "you need to see me, I'm sick" appointment. They booked me in for the next day and the visit was not pleasant. My lung function dropped to a new low of 0.69 FEV1, and since I had just finished oral antibiotics the doctor decided it was time to bring out the big guns: IV antibiotics in this case. She wanted to admit me immediately. Since there were no beds available in the hospital, after waiting for five hours, she gave me the option to either go to the emergency room and be admitted there (although the lack of beds meant I would be in the general emergency section all night with germs everywhere), or go home for the night and hope there was a bed in the morning. I chose the latter.

I ended up getting a bed in the respiratory wing. It was quite the change from being admitted to a general wing in Halifax where few of the nurses seemed to know anything about CF medications or treatments. The nurses at St. Mike's let me sleep in (yes!), administer my own medication, and were just all-around wonderful. Even the food, while not awesome, was as good as mass-produced food could be. The best part about the stay was that they had an optional CF menu from which I could order chips and chocolate bars for snacks.

That hospital stay was the first time I had been in a room where it was obvious that people had spent a long time and then died. Having a picture in the room that was "donated in memory of John Smith" just hammers home the idea that John Smith probably died in that bed. I know that almost every hospital room has had people die in it, but I wasn't a fan of the reminder. The other difference from the general wings that surprised me was all the decals on the walls. Nurses in general wards seem to frown upon patients sticking anything to the walls. In this wing no one seemed to care. I had a room with bamboo stickers, hearts, and endless inspirational phrases telling me to Live, Love, and Laugh. It was clear that someone had spent a lot of time in that room. But I did not appreciate it. I hate pointless inspirational phrases. I hate being told to "dance in the rain" or that "you can't control the storm but you can adjust your sails." These platitudes do nothing except annoy me. I find humour in most situations, which I think is why I have coped so well with all my health issues. I know some people find comfort in inspiring quotes and mantras, but they aren't for me.

Back at the hospital, I got a peripherally inserted central catheter (PICC) line inserted the day after admission, which was a huge relief as it meant that the antibiotics could be given faster than through an IV. The nurses can also draw blood from the line which meant less poking overall. My veins are always happier when I have a PICC line because it means they get a break from IVs and needles for blood work. The actual procedure, however, took two tries for the doctor to get the line in my arm; it felt like forever.

During my previous hospitalizations in Halifax, I was always admitted for a solid two or three weeks so I could get a full run of the medication. However, St. Mike's seemed to operate differently. I moved in enough clothes and books to last me weeks, but after a few days, my sputum samples were tested again. It turned out that one of the bugs I had been growing was no longer there so the main iv antibiotic I was on was pointless. The second iv drug I was taking was shown to be just as effective as an oral medication (many medications are not, as the body doesn't absorb them as well from the stomach, compared to being pumped directly into the bloodstream). The doctor ordered me some pills and just like that—five days after I was admitted—I was cleared to go home.

Of course, I was happy to be home because I never sleep or relax well in the hospital, but it was the first time I had left a hospital admission feeling as though I hadn't been "fixed." They didn't discharge me because I was doing better, they discharged me because there was no point in being admitted to take some pills. Even though I was doing slightly better than when I first went in, I certainly wasn't back to my baseline energy-wise. I was afraid I might never again return to that baseline.

Being home also made me afraid that I might overexert myself, which would put me right back in the hospital. It was easy to do at home because I would always want to do something other than sit on the couch. I needed a shock collar that zapped whenever I decided I was going to do something too active. Me: "Let's go to the zoo tomorrow!" *Zap*! "Ah! I guess I'll sit here and read instead."

To my surprise, the fear of overdoing it never came to fruition. Instead I only felt like lying in bed all day. After three days of that, I forced myself to go outside and visit my cousins for the last swim of the summer. I felt better once I was there, but again crashed upon returning home. I kept wondering if I was finally experiencing the depression that the social worker had warned me about. If I was depressed, then I wanted to get myself on antidepressants so I could feel better. I knew that five days of feeling tired and lethargic did not count as being medically depressed, but I wanted a reason to account for why I felt like shit other than, "Because this is how your body works now." I was hoping it was just a side effect of the medication and that I would feel better once I finished it. I was also worried that I was trapped in a cycle where the medication made me tired, and being tired all the time made me depressed, which made me tired. Part of what made that time challenging was that I felt my hope slipping away, the hope of my "second chance" and that I would return to a life in which I was healthy and could travel the world. Instead of any of that, my health was slowly declining, my lungs weren't responding to medication, and I felt as though, eventually, I was going to run out of bottoms to hit before the new lungs I was promised ever arrived.

Honestly, when I was first listed, I didn't have full confidence that the transplant was going to happen or that it would even help that much if I did have it. When I started seeing how much it changed people's lives, I started getting hopeful, dreaming of all the things I would do once I got my lungs: hike, run, bike, travel, jump, walk up a flight of stairs without getting winded, swim, and so on. I was starting to imagine all the "could bes" and "what ifs," but at that point in September, when they sent me home to our apartment, a transplant felt more like a fantasy and my hopes would be dashed. It wasn't even the length of the wait that was the most discouraging, it was more that the duration of the wait never changed. I was no closer to getting new lungs one day than I was a month prior or would be a month in the future because it's not a "first come, first served" system.

I was feeling depressed, but part of me knew I could get through it. While it was not a pleasant two weeks, it was part of the "down" of the ups and downs that happen when one is chronically ill. I don't think there is any way to avoid those "downs," and the best thing sometimes is to just let them happen while recognizing that they won't last forever.

I had a clinic appointment the following week. I went in hopeful that my lungs had improved because I was feeling a little better and everything had been going okay at physiotherapy. I left feeling horrible. My lung function was unchanged. The good news was that they didn't admit me. The bad news was the only reason I wasn't admitted was that I'd previously had an allergic reaction to the only IV medication they wanted to try, and there were no other options.

Not reacting to treatment is scary. Basically, my lungs had defeated everything science had to offer and the doctors were running out of medication options. While at that point, treatment was more about keeping me alive until the transplant rather than fixing my lungs, it would've been reassuring if my lungs had improved a bit, because I was on enough antibiotics to take down a horse (okay, maybe a slight exaggeration). I was scared that if I got another cold—or worse, the flu or pneumonia—I wouldn't have anything left to fight it off. Turns out that it's true you should be careful what you wish for: before I moved to Toronto to be listed (when I was still imagining getting my lungs at the "average" eight-month mark and moving back home after one year), I said I wished it were possible for me to wait until my lungs were at their absolute last breath and get the transplant then, when I 100% knew there was no chance of living much longer. I was getting to that point and it was terrifying.

I went in for another clinic visit the first week of October, a week after my terrible appointment. The results were slightly better: my lung function had improved up to a FEV1 of 0.77, which meant the drugs were finally working, if only slightly. I also talked to the psychologist and told him all my woes about feeling unmotivated and hopeless since being admitted to the hospital. In the end, he just repeated what everyone else had been telling me: "You're under a lot of stress and waiting is hard. It's normal to have days or weeks when you don't feel like yourself." Even though it was nothing new, it was reassuring to talk to someone removed from the situation and outside of my friends and family (who basically *had* to tell me that I was doing okay).

After that visit, I started feeling more like myself. I went to some pottery drop-in classes. Isaiah and I went on a road trip to see the fall colours, and we visited some family. On October 8, 2014, I hit the one-year waiting mark, which felt like a significant date. One year of silence. I started to think that maybe they had forgotten about me.

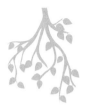

8

HITTING ROCK BOTTOM

OCTOBER TO NOVEMBER 23, 2014

had a good three weeks in October, feeling more energetic and finally getting rid of the side effects from the antibiotics (nausea, bowel issues, etc.), when I went to my weekly clinic appointment to discover that my lung function had dropped down to 19%, or FEV1 of 0.67. Surprise! I knew that the bump from the medication wouldn't last long, but I had been hoping that I would have a good six to eight weeks before it wore off, especially since I was still on one heavy-duty oral antibiotic at the time (that was clearly doing nothing). I had been excited to be finally responding to the medication. Clearly, that outlook was premature. I did not go into that appointment expecting my lung function to have dropped to the lowest it had ever been, without even noticing. How did I not feel that my lung function was down to 19%? I'm still perplexed by this.

I knew my lung function had declined as I had needed more oxygen while walking and felt more short of breath, but I didn't expect it to be at the lowest it had ever been. It's eerie to have your body crap out on you when you don't feel symptomatic. It's like you have no connection to your body and don't know what's happening internally. The decline made sense in hindsight (that's why I had been feeling more short of breath when walking to the bus), but it was shocking at the time. I think it just speaks to how well the body can adjust and compensate when the physical decline is gradual.

For that visit the doctor wasn't encouraging. She had a lot of dispiriting remarks such as, "Your lung function numbers are freaking me out"; "I don't know what medication to give you anymore"; and, "We're stuck between a rock and a hard place." The plan was to be sent home on some new antibiotics, and once my sputum culture report was completed, I would go back into the hospital for some iv antibiotics. Unfortunately, I couldn't go back on the antibiotic that had worked a few weeks prior if I wanted to keep my kidneys (and I did). The side effects from that medication are strong and tend to destroy other organs. The doctors don't like to keep people on this antibiotic for longer than a month at a time, and my month was up. I was running out of new antibiotics to try.

On October 25, I was back in St. Mike's for a stay. I was on iv antibiotics twice a day, which wasn't too bad. The nurse warned me about the medication causing serious nausea. For the first few hours I thought I might be okay. Then in the span of fifteen minutes, I went from feeling fine to wanting to curl up and vomit. I was also told that I was now officially on the status two "high priority" list as of the previous day. This was news to me. I thought I had been told during my September hospitalization that I was being switched to high priority permanently; apparently I had misinterpreted, "We'll talk with the doctors at TGH about bumping you up to high priority," for, "You're in the high priority group."

The most frustrating part about the status listing was that my CF doctor had emailed the transplant doctors to confirm my status only to be sent the response, "But she doesn't need to be status two, she has been doing so well at physio." The CF doctor thankfully answered with, "That is because she is a determined person and not because her lungs are any good." My CF doctor managed to convince the transplant team that because my lungs were barely responding to the medication, I was much sicker than I appeared.

It seemed as though the transplant doctors based their determination of "high priority" more on how a person functions day-to-day and at physiotherapy than on the actual lung function number. Someone could have a higher lung function than me (and some people waiting probably did) but would require a wheelchair or have more physical limitations. As I've said, lung function drop affects everyone differently. So in that regard, it's practical that they look at how people are physically functioning rather than bumping people up when they hit a predetermined number. It makes sense; it's just frustrating when you're the person with horrible lungs who can somehow still function relatively well, so you are overlooked.

The lesson I want to pass on for anyone reading this who is starting the lung transplant program is that if your lungs are not responding to treatment but you aren't status two, don't try very hard at physiotherapy. Well, do, because physiotherapy certainly helps recovery, but don't try super-hard during walk tests. Or pretend to be more physically weak than you are and work out for real at a different gym. Or complain a lot to the physiotherapists. Truthfully, don't do any of that, but make sure to tell the physiotherapists how you feel without trying to put a positive spin on life like I often did. Instead of saying, "I'm fine," I should've been saying, "I felt sick yesterday and threw up this morning, but at this moment, I'm fine because I'm not currently vomiting. So maybe I'm fine? I'm not fine. I threw up this morning."

I was discharged from St. Mike's on October 29. The doctors really didn't like keeping me in the hospital. My lung function had improved marginally, and since I wasn't symptomatic and my sputum cultures showed just the regular respiratory bugs, the doctor said she had no real argument to keep me hospitalized. I was once again sent home on oral antibiotics which made me feel terrible and I spent several days trying not to vomit. The temptation to quit treatment gets stronger as it takes a greater toll on the body. It's a horrible necessity that often the medication makes one feel worse than the condition. However, it's usually worth it on the other side.

My goal to stay out of the hospital for the month of November lasted an entire nine days. On the Wednesday after pottery class, I felt unusually short of breath walking to the subway. And "more than usual" for me seemed significant. It was beyond my usual fatigue. I felt as though I was having an asthma attack: my lungs were seizing and I struggled to get my breath back. I hadn't felt that way for years.

While I may have been officially diagnosed with asthma as a child (there is some debate in my family over this), and it is a common secondary disease for people with CF, it's not usually something the doctors pay much attention to as they can't do more for treatment than continue the aerosol masks and puffers. In retrospect, I think I may have gotten short of breath while I was carrying a box of pottery at the time, started panicking about my shortness of breath, and then had an anxiety attack. Either way, I had to keep taking significant rest breaks in order to get home. It was terrible and more of a struggle than I had experienced in years. Once I was home and had pumped up my oxygen a bit, I felt better and chalked it up to a weird incident.

I attended physiotherapy Thursday and Friday that week, and while I felt more shortness of breath than usual and my oxygen levels were down slightly, I still felt okay overall. So I carried on. I passed it off due to the cold weather and simply being tired— it's remarkable what the mind can rationalize. On Saturday, I felt short of breath simply walking around the apartment and then my stomach revolted. When I threw up my "thirteen-month wait" celebration meal, I knew it was time to call the doctor.

The doctor on call that night informed me that the respiratory beds were full so I had to be admitted through the emergency department. He said it was okay to wait until Sunday morning so I could have one last sleep in my bed. If I had known how long it would be before I slept in that bed again, I may never have gotten out. I showed up at the emergency department early Sunday morning, told them my problems, and spent the day waiting around for a bed on a floor. I had always dreaded being admitted through the emergency department and had avoided it at all possible cost, but it turned out to be okay. Upon arrival, I was immediately whisked off to a stretcher in the ward so I didn't have to be in the general waiting room with the random people who were coughing and sneezing. I spent the afternoon speculating about the diagnoses of the other patients while knitting and listening to podcasts.

The doctors couldn't figure out why I was suddenly so short of breath, and although they believed me, they wanted to test my lung function for themselves. When I was finally tested, it was surprisingly good news: my lung function was up! My body no longer made sense to me, and I felt so disconnected from my lungs. How was it that I felt so terrible, yet my lungs had jumped up to a FEV1 of 0.82? How could I feel good a month ago when my lung function was the lowest ever? It was all disconcerting. However, clearly the antibiotic was working, which was good news, even if I couldn't feel it.

The other shocking improvement was that my oxygen levels had returned to around the baseline from months prior. The respirologist took me for a walk around the hallway and said I should decrease my levels to one litre at rest and three litres for exertion (I had been using two litres at rest and four litres for exertion). The team wanted to keep me on the lowest possible oxygen setting. If there is too much oxygen artificially pumped into the body, then carbon dioxide can build up because the lungs aren't strong enough to transfer it out, and this can cause poisoning. I preferred not be to poisoned with oxygen, although it occurred to me that if I did die that way, it would be ironic and I wanted everyone to make highly inappropriate jokes at my funeral.

None of this explained why I was so short of breath while doing basic activities like walking down the hall or showering. The respiratory therapist (RT) tried to explain that when the lungs are severely scarred, sometimes people feel short of breath because all the body and brain can do is focus on breathing. That made sense, but he couldn't explain why it happened so fast. I should've been able to do cartwheels in the hall with a FEV1 of 0.82 or, you know, shower without feeling like I might fall over. I asked him if it was something I just needed to push through and live with from now on. He responded yes. And as

I had been told it seemed a million times in the past thirteen months, he repeated, "The stronger you are going into surgery, the better you'll do post-op."

It looked like I just needed to deal with it.

I could do that.

With my lung function increasing, they talked about kicking me out (my phrasing) of the hospital even though I was still short of breath while doing anything remotely physical. I didn't think that they would discharge me as I was so symptomatic and felt terrible. I was tired all the time and I just wanted them to fix me. I never thought I would reach the point where I would advocate staying longer in the hospital, but I felt that maybe if I got a full dose of IV antibiotics, I would be in a better position upon discharge. Instead, the doctor told me to try giving myself some time off oxygen, despite the fact that I still felt short of breath. It felt strange to not be wearing oxygen all the time. I had imagined that it would be a relief to get rid of the nasal prongs, but instead I kept feeling phantom tubing. I either felt like I was still wearing it and would go to move the line when I walked around the room, or I felt like something was missing.

I continued to feel exhausted and short of breath even though my oxygen saturation was stable. A different RT explained that when someone has an infection in the lower lobes, it's harder for the blood to get oxygenated so the body desaturates. However, if the infection is more in the upper lobes (like they thought mine was), then the blood still gets oxygen (as when you're standing, gravity draws it to the bottom of the lungs). The shortness of breath continues because the body is still struggling to get air into the upper lobes. It made sense when he explained it. It was a different explanation from the first RT's but it seemed to account for my shortness of breath.

Two days later, when I got a pass from the hospital to walk to the St. Lawrence Market, my lungs seemed to seize while outside. It was the first time I had walked anywhere without oxygen in a very long time and the wind and cold shocked my lungs. My oxygen levels dropped and my heart rate spiked, despite the fact that I was walking at turtle speed and taking frequent breaks. It was frustrating, and when I returned to the hospital, I ended up back on the oxygen for the rest of the day as my lungs took a long time to recover.

Mom and Dad were visiting, so the next day, Mom and I went off to a drop-in pottery class. This time we cabbed it to give my lungs a break. I barely walked at all that day and when I did, I walked at my turtle speed. Still, I continued to get short of breath. I was disheartened and returned to the hospital to complain to the doctor that they needed to fix me. The doctor's new theory as to why I still couldn't breathe was that I had serious inflammation. Her theory was that I had a build-up of stale air in my lungs due to my not exhaling completely. The solution: I needed to start a new anti-inflammatory.

I said goodbye to my parents, who flew back home, and on Monday I met the new attending doctor for that week. The new doctor had his own theories on why I was so short of breath. While the doctors all work together, they all seem to have their own approach for testing and treatment. So I wasn't surprised when, that same morning, I was whisked off for an ECG with no explanation. In the afternoon, I was whisked off again for a CT scan. It was the gross dye one where they inject dye into the bloodstream that both burns and makes me feel as though I'm peeing for about five seconds. (I don't actually pee, it's just feels like I am. It's a random side effect from the dye but happens every time.)

After the Monday tests, the doctor told me the good and bad news. The good news was that they now knew for sure why I was short of breath despite my "high" lung function. Every theory I had heard from the RTs and doctors had been wrong. They finally had the reason, which was the bad news: it was because

I had a pulmonary embolism (a.k.a. a blood clot) in my lung. The doctors didn't know where the clot came from, although my PICC line was a suspect.

Having a pulmonary embolism filled me with dread. A clot is much more serious and terrifying than an infection or inflammation because nothing can be done other than to wait for it to break down while feeling paranoid that it's going to travel to the heart or brain. After that news, I had ultrasounds done of my legs and arms to make sure there were no more clots floating around. They started me on blood thinners to prevent any new ones from forming and to help the clot dissolve. All the IV antibiotics were stopped as I clearly had no infection. But soon after stopping them, I suddenly started getting fevers.

I continued to feel worse over the next few days. My fever continued so I was restarted on the antibiotics to give my lungs extra support. This caused me to feel nauseous all the time. I was pumped full of saline to make sure I stayed hydrated, but the team didn't want to do any further interventions. The doctors thought the fever and chills had been caused by the flu as I had started to develop muscle aches and a sore throat on top of everything.

And just like that, my remaining energy was zapped. All of the medication, plus the fever, took everything out of me. I found that I needed more support than ever simply going to the bathroom or getting food out of the little fridge in my room. I slept most of the time and would go from freezing to hot in minutes. The nurses weren't supposed to give me Tylenol unless my temperature reached a certain number, but since I would get chills before I reached that point, I would buzz them to try and get medication early, before the chills escalated. A few nurses would take pity on my shivering state and give me Tylenol early, but most of them made me wait until my temperature reached the critical number because they wanted to make sure I actually had a fever. It was a miserable few days.

On November 21, 2014, my flu swab returned negative so that was ruled out as the cause of my fevers. I was short of breath all the time so I was started on a Bilevel Positive Airway Pressure machine (more commonly known as the BiPap machine) "when needed," which helped. Although I resisted using it at first, as soon as I started wearing it, I never wanted to take it off. The nurses lectured me on only using it "when necessary," because it weakens the lungs if a person is on it too long: it causes the lungs to start losing whatever muscles they had. I started wearing the BiPap while sleeping and after walking anywhere, and it made me much more comfortable.

The ICU staff started following me because I was doing so poorly on the respiratory floor. Although the ICU team didn't recommend any new interventions, they kept checking my status to see how I was progressing. Their theory about the temperatures was that my PICC line was infected, and they wanted to pull it out. As it was the only way I was getting medication, the nurses and I wanted it kept in to avoid them having to find veins for IVs.

On November 23, my parents flew back to Toronto, full of concern. Nothing seemed to be improving even though the doctors kept reassuring me that they had everything under control. My parents were understandably worried, and I was in no position to tell them whether they should visit or stay home on the chance that I would improve. In that situation, it's difficult to gauge how sick you are. I remained optimistic that my health would improve while facing the reality that I wasn't getting better. I knew it was bad when I was slightly hungry but didn't have the energy to get out of bed to get food from my fridge two feet away. There was no more sugar-coating it: I was dying. It was good that Mom and Dad jumped on a plane because the next day, I got The Call.

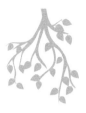

9

THE CALL

The difference between how the Almighty Transplant Manual described The Call and what happened in my case was extreme. The manual said I would get The Call and would then have to stop eating and get myself to the hospital as soon as possible. The manual stated that calling an ambulance is the last resort and strongly frowned upon. I'm not sure why anyone would call an ambulance as their first option because in the end it would cost much more than a cab. Once I arrived at the hospital, I would go to the floor (during the day) or the emergency department (at night). I would have an ECG, x-ray, blood tests, and IVs would be inserted. This could take three to four hours, and at any point in this process, the surgery could be called off. There are a lot of false calls (a.k.a. "dry runs") while the team runs tests on the donor lungs. Sometimes they find an infection or bruising, which means that both lungs may not be viable and then the surgery cannot proceed.

If the surgery proved viable, my family could visit me in the transplant ICU immediately afterward, even though I'd be on crazy amounts of pain medications, connected to numerous tubes and machines, and I'd be delirious—great family bonding time. After I could breathe on my own (which might take a few days or weeks), I would go to the Multi-Organ Transplant Step-Down Unit, also known as the "Acute Care Unit." When I graduated from that unit, I would go to the Multi-Organ Transplant Unit, where I would be in intensive physiotherapy, learn about my anti-rejection medications, and recover until I was ready to be discharged.

I soon learned that what is written in the Almighty Transplant Manual is based more on an "ideal situation," and that while it describes how The Call is supposed to go, it doesn't work out that way for many people.

On Monday, November 24, 2014, the day of The Call, Mom and Dad arrived back in Toronto and spent the day at the hospital. I felt like shit, to be frank, and didn't have energy to do anything. Before, when people were visiting I could usually rally to get out of the hospital for a short while, but this time I could barely leave the bed. I managed to drink some Booster Juice and tried to put as much of a positive spin on things as I could. Now there was no denying that I wasn't getting any better. I continued to get fevers and chills and felt as though my body was shutting down. Because it was.

That evening as I was doing my aerosol mask, two nurses came into my room. I sensed something was happening because there were rarely two nurses working together, and they seemed almost giddy. They informed me that they had just received a call from the TGH and that there were lungs for me: I was finally going to get my transplant! I was dazed. What were they talking about? Why was the Toronto General calling them? The manual said they would be calling me. The nurses repeated the information, a bit less excited this time, saying that since the team at TGH knew I was at St. Mike's, they decided to bypass me and inform my doctors and nurses first. I was to spend that night at St. Mike's and then be transferred to the TGH the next morning to begin the process.

It's hard to describe the feeling I had when I was told I had been called. It was a kaleidoscope of emotions: anxiety, relief, but mostly disbelief and exhaustion. I didn't know how to feel so I did what I do best when overwhelmed, I shut down my emotions for a while. I'm not exactly good at outwardly expressing my emotions in the first place, but it seems the lack of emotion wasn't what the nurses were expecting. They seemed somewhat deflated when I responded with a stoic, "Okay, cool." I'm not sure if they expected me to start jumping up and down in excitement or burst into tears, but I had no energy for either. I'm not sure I would've reacted any differently even if I had had more energy. One of them said something like, "Well, aren't you going to call someone to let them know?" Of course I was going to call someone, but I just needed a minute for the shock to wear off first. I was also still doing my aerosol mask, which meant talking was challenging. The nurses seemed perplexed by my lack of apparent excitement and eventually left after I reassured them that I would indeed contact my family. I just didn't want to do it with them hovering over me.

I finished my aerosol mask and then had to weigh whether it was worth being off the BiPap machine to call people, as I couldn't talk with the machine running but couldn't breathe comfortably with it off. I eventually called Isaiah and told him that I got The Call and to be at the hospital for 6:00 A.M. to pack up my room so he could be there when they came to transfer me. I also called Amy but all she heard were the breathing noises of the BiPap machine and my voice saying, "Got. Call. Lungs. Tomorrow." Since talking on the phone didn't work, I hung up on her and just texted instead. She then called my parents who were on the subway heading to stay with their friends in Richmond Hill. Mom had twenty missed calls from Amy when she got cell service again.

When I had imagined getting The Call, I pictured calling everyone I knew to have long meaningful conversations with them in case I died during the surgery. I figured I would have lots of time while waiting for everything to go through. I imagined crying with excitement on the phone and telling all my friends and family how much I loved them and how much they meant to me. What I didn't picture was that I would already be sitting in a hospital room, not having the energy to do much else than focus on my breathing. No long meaningful conversations happened; no, "If I die tomorrow, I hope you know how much I love you," talks. Instead everyone got a text saying (yes, I sent the same text to everyone), "I got The Call!!!!! Timeline: Stay at St. Mike's tonight, travel by ambulance to Toronto General at 6:00 A.M., start pre-op madness, hopefully be in surgery by tomorrow night!! Holy F, it's finally (maybe) happening!! I can't chat on the phone as I'm on the BiPap but Amy will update the blog continuously as we go."

I think that was the excitement the nurses were looking for. It was easier to express in text. The shock wore off and fear of what was about to happen settled in. I didn't think I would sleep at all that night, but somehow I managed to get a few hours' rest.

I don't remember much of Tuesday, November 25, 2014. It is all a bit hazy, but between what I can remember and what people have described, I'll give it my best shot to piece events together.

I was up bright and early on the Tuesday morning. Isaiah and my parents showed up for the 6:00 A.M. transfer to the TGH. The paramedics transferred me to the other hospital. Unfortunately, they had to take me off the BiPap machine for the ride. I was put on regular oxygen, strapped to the transfer board, and away we went. Isaiah rode in the ambulance with me and (I think) my parents took a cab. Upon arriving at the TGH, they had a bed waiting for me in the transplant general admittance floor where I managed to sleep.

I woke up from my nap feeling short of breath, so when the RT came in, I asked if it was possible to be put back on the BiPap machine—it had been working so well for me at St. Mike's. She responded that they weren't able to use the BiPap as it was considered too much of a medical intervention for the level of care on that floor. If they were going to use it then I would have to be transferred to a different floor. I had no problem with that; I didn't care what floor I was on, but no one else seemed to want me to make that move. She brought a high-flow oxygen machine and cranked it up despite my protests that while I liked the BiPap machine, I didn't need that much oxygen and was on a lower flow at the other hospital. She ignored me, and since I did feel better with oxygen shooting into my brain I managed to nap again.

Back in the Maritimes, Amy and David were trying to decide if they should come up that day or wait to see if the surgery went ahead. I was adamant that there was no point in them flying up until I knew whether or not it was a false call, but they didn't listen to me. Later Amy said that she decided she needed to fly up ASAP because even if I didn't make it into surgery, it was clear that I was going to need to be on a ventilator soon. She felt they should visit me before I reached that point.

I awoke when a doctor came in to put Xs on my chest as an indication of what procedure was happening. For some reason, I found that absolutely hilarious. I would hope that they would switch out both lungs without needing Xs to remember. Better safe than sorry, I suppose.

I had another nap and when I woke up, I knew something wasn't right. I couldn't focus on anything and my body felt weird. It was as though I was floating and there was a disconnect between me and the rest of the world. I could see people and hear them through a fog, but I couldn't focus my eyes on anything. I couldn't form words to describe the feeling other than to say that "It wasn't right, I can't focus on anything, and my brain is broken." I repeated over and over that my brain was broken and that I needed Isaiah to fix me. It was hard for me to even explain that much.

I started to completely panic that I would be in this hazy, in-between-worlds stage forever and kept telling Isaiah to snap me out of it just like the people did in all the podcasts I had listened to. (Some context: I had just listened to a Radiolab podcast about a woman who kept talking to her daughter who was in a coma, despite the doctors saying that the daughter would never wake up. But then she did.) I remember repeating that if the podcast people could snap their loved ones out of a coma, then he could snap me out of whatever was happening to me. He kept responding that those experiences are rare and that he wasn't in a podcast story. My parents and Isaiah, clearly concerned, rang the nurse, telling them that I was acting strangely.

The nurse lowered my oxygen levels and rang the RT, who kept telling me that everything was okay. I insisted that everything wasn't okay, I felt weird, my brain was broken, and please, for the love of God, fix it. Eventually, someone thought to check my blood gas levels. Turns out they were extremely high. My lungs weren't able to extract all the oxygen being pushed into my body and I had built up carbon dioxide. The stupid high-flow oxygen machine was poisoning me. After all my fears about getting poisoned, it had come true.

I don't remember much after that. I'm told that they eventually transferred me to the floor where BiPap machines were allowed and then reduced my oxygen flow—all it took was being poisoned and ranting incoherently about podcasts. I drifted in and out of consciousness/coherence for the rest of the day. Apparently, at one point, a resident told me that they weren't sure if the transplant was going to happen as the lungs were not a perfect match. The team was working hard but they weren't positive that they could make them fit. The resident said that if it didn't happen, it looked like they would have to put me on a ventilator because I was struggling so hard to breathe. Mom says that when he said this, I started crying and begged for it not to happen. I don't remember any of that conversation.

At 4:00 A.M. on Wednesday, November 26, 2014, they wheeled me off to surgery for my double-lung transplant. Mom says she was never so happy to see me taken away for a procedure. My family didn't know if I would come back alive, but they knew I had no chance if I stayed in my current state much longer. All I remember is waking up in an elevator with medical people around me, and I'm not even sure if that was on my way to surgery or from the previous day's transfer. I woke up again in a surgery room with more medical people around me before passing out again. That's all I remember until I woke up four days later, dazed and confused, convinced I was still poisoned.

PART III

RECOVERY IN THE HOSPITAL

NOVEMBER 27, 2014 TO JANUARY 2015

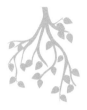

10

ON THE OTHER
SIDE OF SURGERY

'm told that after they wheeled me in for surgery, Isaiah went
home to get some sleep after being up all night. I had told all of
my family to go home as there was no point in everyone being
exhausted, but my parents didn't listen to me. Mom and Dad
stayed at the hospital to wait it out. It was a long wait. Twelve
hours later, I was out of surgery but on an extracorporeal mem-
brane oxygenation (ECMO) machine. An ECMO is a device that
is connected to the body by a central line that pulls blood into
a machine that exchanges the gases before pumping it back.
This mimics a lung. The ECMO has a number of high-risk complications, such as stroke and heart failure, so it's only used in

life-saving situations. It was too early to say that the surgery went well considering that the ECMO machine was keeping me alive, but at least I was alive. Although the surgeon had to cut down the lungs for my body and I had some bleeding, the transplant was declared a success. The doctor told my family to expect me to need an extended recovery time due to the ECMO machine; I had to be kept sedated longer than usual to give my body time to recover and accept the new lungs.

Amy, David, and Cindy (David's wife) made it to Toronto the night of my surgery, beating a November snowstorm. They came to see me in the transplant ICU the next morning (November 27). Mom warned them many times how terrible I looked and to be prepared for all the medical equipment around my body. I was still connected, via a line in my neck, to the ECMO machine, which was transferring blood in and out of my body.

The next day was a problem for David because he walked in when the nurses were doing plasma transfusions. That meant there were even more lines of blood than had been there the day before. Most people are not big fans of seeing blood, but David has always been extra sensitive. Amy said the tubes full of my blood whirring around were too much for him. He turned ghost-white and Amy was positive he was going to pass out. To avoid both of us in the ICU, he lay down in the waiting room and then she forced him to go to the hospital's Starbucks to inhale some coffee fumes and drink some tea as a break from the normal hospital smells. Sorry, bro, for almost making you faint!

The doctor allowed me to wake up a little that day, not that I remember, but apparently I gave out hugs to everyone before panicking about life. I was promptly put back to sleep to let my body rest. It was an emotional day for the family, who now believed that I might pull through. The surgeon was optimistic that I would be okay because I was doing better than he expected and my ventilator was able to be weaned down a little. He also told my family that the big delay between the actual call and the surgery was because they struggled to get the set of lungs to work for me. They knew there was only a slim chance that I would live long enough for another pair to become available, so they did everything they could to make these ones work for me.

On November 28, I was taken off the ECMO but then had some bleeding in one of my lungs and had to go back into the operating room to get it drained. The surgeon managed to fix the problem and reassured my family that it was a common occurrence. Apparently, since my original lungs were so bad, more or less just scar tissue from all my previous infections, they were hard to remove. The scar tissue can, apparently, cause bleeding later with the new lungs as the body cavity is still struggling to recover. The bleeding may have also been caused by the ECMO machine as it thins the blood, making one more prone to bleeding. After being removed from the ECMO, I was finally breathing on my own with the aid of pressure support from a ventilator and oxygen. The next day, I was able to open my eyes when someone spoke to me, and they started weaning me off the pain medication so I would slowly wake up. They also started to feed me through a nasal (NG) tube.

November 30 is when I woke up convinced I was still poisoned and not knowing what was happening. The last thing I remembered coherently was being poisoned, so this was a logical conclusion to me. I didn't know that I had had the transplant. Although I could barely remember the day before the surgery, I was waking up four days after the surgery; it felt like I had lost five days. I was so mixed-up. Waking up alone in a dark hospital room after being poisoned is not something I would recommend to anyone.

After the nurse assured me that I did not have carbon dioxide poisoning, although my levels were a bit high when I woke up (I guess being paranoid is a good thing), and that I had had the surgery, I was relieved but still confused. I was on a ridiculous amount of pain medication, but being unaware you're on pain medication that is messing up your brain makes for some interesting thoughts. Turns out those people that I had seen hiding in the hallway, yeah, those weren't actually people. That was just my brain on drugs. They also weren't selling tacos. I would drift in and out of consciousness but without realizing it, so I would hear nurses mentioning something about me, fall asleep (without knowing), and wake up assuming they were still talking about me.

Sometime on the morning of November 30, the physiotherapist showed up to get me out of bed for the first time, and suddenly the x-ray technicians appeared to take a chest x-ray. Once they had forced me up into a sitting position to take the x-ray (I had no muscles to move anything, I couldn't even lift my head off the pillow), I was exhausted. The physiotherapist pulled me into a sitting position again, and I thought I was going to pass out. I sat on the side of the bed with someone holding me for a solid five minutes before my head stopped spinning. Then I tried to stand up. You know when you've been marathon-watching Netflix and you suddenly realize you have to pee so you try to sprint to the bathroom before the next show loads but realize that your legs are asleep and you kind of fall over? That happened. I'm not sure what happens to most people, but I fell over. Thankfully, the physiotherapist caught me and kind of threw me over the stand-up walker to support my weight and forced me to stand for several hours. Okay, it was only maybe a minute in total, but it felt like hours. It was exhausting. The physiotherapist had said she wanted me to go for a walk, but because I almost passed out while standing, she quickly changed her mind and had me sit back in bed, saying she would be back the next day and every single day afterward until I could walk out of the department.

Amy arrived shortly after the physiotherapist left. I was surprised to see her, as at that point, I didn't know she had flown up. She was pleased to see me awake and informed me the family was in the waiting room, waiting for me to come around. It's always awkward to visit someone who can't talk or communicate in any way, but she seemed to be able to do it well. The nurse got me a letter board, which helped somewhat.

For those who don't know, letter boards are ridiculously hard to use. It seems like it should be straightforward: it's a board with the alphabet where you point at the letter you want. Pretty easy. Except that no one uses them when everything is working at 100% capacity. At the time when my eyes couldn't focus (plus I didn't have my glasses for the first day), my brain was muddled from the pain medication and my hands shook, it was hard to remember how the alphabet went, how anything was spelled, and how to form sentences. Also, people try to do you a favour by guessing the rest of the word, and as a result, they often forgot the first letters. "W-H-A-T. What are we doing? What are we eating? What are we up to? What is happening? What was that you had said?" I wanted to scream at them to be patient and stop jumping in, but of course if I could have done that, we wouldn't have needed the letter board. I would also confuse the *B*s and *P*s or the *I*s and *L*s, which didn't help anyone guess the word I was trying to spell. I was thankful when my eyes focused and my hand stopped shaking enough so that I could switch to scrawling out messages on paper.

I had heard the nurses talking about the Jian Ghomeshi situation, so I had Amy fill me in on what had happened since I stopped remembering events. The rest of the family visited later in the day and showed me the last pottery pieces they had picked up for me. Because only two people were allowed in the room at one time, everyone had to rotate their visits. It was nice, in a way, that visitors were limited so I wasn't swamped with seeing everyone at once, but it also meant that I would often have to repeat the same thing when someone new came in.

The transplant ICU is one-to-one nursing care and the hospital bed is placed in the centre of the room with all the necessary equipment in it. The nurse sits outside of the room and there is a window so the patient can be watched at all times. Because it's a one-to-one ratio, there are no call bells as the nurse is supposed to be ready whenever you may need anything. Of course there is usually someone on break, which means it's a two-to-one ratio and then one patient ends up being under-attended for a period of time. There were many times when I tried to get a nurse's attention but couldn't because I had no way of drawing attention to myself. I couldn't talk, and while I could wave my arm around a little, I had to take breaks because the movement was exhausting. This meant that there was no chance of getting their attention if I had anything with which I needed immediate help.

Lying in bed, not being able to move, is a terrible experience. I had no muscle mass and it didn't help that the bed was an "air bed," which is top quality and the best for preventing bed sores but didn't help my comfort. It was uncomfortable when the nurses rotated me, and as someone used to sleeping on her side or stomach, sleeping on my back all the time was hard. I could pass out for a while but found it hard to get back to sleep once I woke up. Once they reduced my hallucination-causing pain medication, I found I was more and more uncomfortable but unable to do anything to make it better. Since I couldn't move, I was reliant on other people for everything. It improved somewhat when I got my phone, some magazines, and knitting, and I was able to entertain myself and keep everything on my side table. The problem was when medical professionals came in to talk, they would usually roll the table away and often forget to roll it back within my reach when they left. I was then stuck with nothing to do as I couldn't call them back into the room and could only make hand gestures or tap on the bed to try to get assistance.

This is your official warning that I'm going to talk about poop for the next few paragraphs. Just skip ahead if you're reading while eating.

The problem with the ICU beds, other than being too soft and uncomfortable, was that they made going to the bathroom impossible. To be fair, it wasn't the bed's fault. I would almost pass out as soon as I stood up, so it wasn't as though I would be walking to a toilet any time soon. Urinating wasn't a problem because I had a catheter, so other than having to move it around once I was finally able to transfer from the bed to a chair, I didn't notice it. Pooping, however, was awful.

Let's be honest, pooping is no joyride to begin with, but as I was being fed 100% liquid calories through my nasal tube, it was all just liquid out as well. And since all of my muscle control was gone, I had absolutely no bowel control. I could sometimes sense when it was about to happen and on the miraculous chance that I got the nurse's attention in time, she would hoist me onto a bedpan. Bedpans are terribly uncomfortable and the body doesn't exactly relax well to poop in the lying position. But if I did relax, sometimes it wouldn't stop. It was all very humiliating and while the nurses kept telling me there was nothing I could do and that it happened to everyone, I felt awful about pooping everywhere. The nurse would usually have to call in an aid to help roll me from side to side afterward to clean everything up, which added exhaustion on top of the humiliation. It helped that I was high on painkillers during most of this.

I got more used to the process after the first few days, but it remains a horrible, panic-inducing memory to this day. I thought maybe writing about it would help me work through the panic, but I'm not sure this strategy is working. Being unable to use the bathroom was one of the major causes of the panic attacks I developed in the hospital. The lack of control as to when or where I could go caused massive stress. Being able to get on a bedpan in time became a real source of anxiety, as often the nurses wouldn't notice me waving. This led to having panic attacks whenever I felt confined in the bed, which was most of the time during the first few weeks post-transplant.

I also started panicking during the physiotherapy sessions because walking around had a tendency to, let's say, loosen everything up. And, boy, did they loosen up one day when I was determined to extend my walk around the nurses' station. I suddenly felt that I had to go and tried to communicate it to the physiotherapist, but as I still couldn't talk and she was busy wheeling in all the equipment with her assistant, she didn't notice. I started panicking, thinking there must be a bathroom I could run into (forgetting momentarily that I could barely walk, let alone run anywhere). I looked at her, wide-eyed, stopped walking, and everything let go. It felt like the lowest moment of my life. I wanted the floor to open up and absorb me so I would never have to see these people again. I sure made everyone work for their money that day. The physiotherapist was kind about it and told me that it happens more than I would think—exercise tends to get everything moving. Nonetheless, for all my following physiotherapy sessions, she made sure that I wore briefs. Overall, it was not a highlight of my life.

Those are enough terrible poop stories, although post-transplant, or after any major surgery, all anyone talks about is poop. It's very important in the recovery process to be pooping properly.

11

BREATHING WITH
NEW LUNGS

The first few days after I officially woke up were fairly quiet. The physiotherapist would arrive in the morning, my family would visit, and doctors just waited for my body to heal. I managed to stand with help from the physiotherapist and shuffle down the hallway a short distance before almost passing out. Progress! I was able to transition from the letter board to shaky writing, which vastly improved my communication. I begged the nurses and doctors to take out my endotracheal tube (ETT) every chance I could. An ETT is the plastic tube inserted through the mouth (or nose) that connects to a mechanical ventilator, which pushes oxygen into the lungs. It can also be connected to a manual bag that someone pumps while mobile. Because it's a tube that leads directly into the lungs, doctors are understandably cautious about allowing people to have water or ice chips with an ETT for fear the liquid will go into the lungs. My mouth was achingly dry. I told the doctors I would just hold the water in my mouth and spit it out but they, rightfully, didn't believe me.

I hadn't done much research about the immediate post-transplant recovery. I had thought it was best to be ignorant about some aspects of the transplant. So getting my lungs suctioned was a huge shock for which I wasn't prepared. The first lung suction (which I received not long after I wakened in the earliest days following the transplant) was terrifying because I had no idea what was happening and, worse, it happened quite suddenly. I had gestured something to the nurse that I thought was a, *What is happening, where am I?* gesture. She had responded by asking if I needed suction. I must've shrugged by way of trying to ask, *What is suctioning?* when she stuck a plastic tube through the ETT and into my lungs.

The nurses use suctioning to remove any phlegm or mucous that builds up post-transplant because the lungs are too weak to cough it up. Suctioning is a weird feeling: it's like someone is tickling your lungs but with a giant plastic tube. I couldn't breathe, it made my lungs seize up, and I felt as though I needed to cough but that action hurt too much. Even if I had had the muscles to cough, I wouldn't have been able to bring anything up due to the ETT in my throat. Suctioning also helps the nurses discern if there is any bleeding in the lungs because if there were, they would suction up gobs of blood. After my first experience, though, once I knew that to expect, the procedure felt okay.

Unexpected procedures aside, breathing itself felt weird. The ventilator was helping my lungs, so while I was technically breathing on my own, I was doing so with a lot of assistance.

It didn't bother me that I now had someone else's lungs; it bothered me that it felt like those lungs were in separate parts. The feeling was strange and difficult to describe, but it was as though I could breathe through my upper lobes, or if I concentrated, through the lower lobes, but I couldn't use both simultaneously. It took a lot of focus to breathe deeply as it felt like I was moving two different muscles. Everyone kept telling me that I would get used to the sensation eventually, but it felt so foreign that I didn't believe them.

In the early afternoon of December 2, the ETT was taken out. The doctors had finally listened to my pleading to remove it. Big mistake. Doctors, never listen to your patients, especially your drug-addled patients! They had decided that since I was on minimal support with the ventilator, they could take out the ETT and put me on the high-flow oxygen to help me breathe. At first I was excited that I was progressing health-wise, until I started to panic. I tried sitting up, thinking it would help me breathe more easily and reduce my anxiety. However, because of the stupid expensive bed that only hindered my efforts, I wasn't able to sit up properly and I continued to panic.

The nurses tried to help: they brought the bed up as high as possible and propped me up with pillows, but it didn't work. The problem was that I didn't have enough strength in my torso to keep myself as upright as I wanted. My family kept up their rotation of visits trying to distract me from panicking and my increasing shortness of breath. The respirologist and RT kept telling me to "not think about it" and "just relax" and a lot of other helpful phrases that have never helped anyone with anxiety since the beginning of time.

I lasted two hours without the ETT before the team conceded that my increasing anxiety wasn't the sole cause of my shortness of breath. At this point, my heart rate had spiked to 190 beats per minute and my oxygen levels crashed to 85%. The doctors gave me medication that lowered my heart rate and another that knocked me out before they shoved the ETT back in my throat and put me back on the ventilator. Okay, so they were more delicate than that, but afterward my throat felt like they had used an ETT made of broken glass. The day was exhausting. Already tired by my short jaunts with the physiotherapist and from trying to communicate with family, that experience put me out for the rest of the day and the following day. It was certainly a "zero steps forward, two steps back" kind of day.

The next day, as the doctors were unhappy with my lack of progress and with the previous day's incident, they ordered a CT scan and ultrasound to investigate why I wasn't able to breathe off the ventilator. The CT scan was a huge ordeal as I had to be wheeled down on my bed with all my equipment. The nursing staff couldn't take the ventilator with them, so my nurse had to "bag me," which meant attaching the ETT to a bag that she pushed every few seconds to pump air into my lungs (like you see on the medical emergency shows). In the actual CT scan room, I had to be transferred with a board from my bed to the CT machine because I didn't have the strength to shuffle myself over. The nurses, CT scan technician, and a porter lifted me up by the sheet of the bed to slide me onto the wooden board. It was uncomfortable. While on the wooden plank, I noticed that my tailbone was feeling bruised. I had to lay perfectly flat for the scan, which was the first time since the surgery I had done that while conscious. I started to panic because it was hard to breathe while lying down. I had a supportive nurse that day who reassured me and then yelled at the technician to work faster.

Once the results were back from the scan, we discovered that one of the reasons for my slow recovery was that I had a pulmonary embolism as well as a clot in the artery by my left shoulder. The team wasn't sure if the clot was from the donor's lungs or the bleeding during or after the surgery, but it explained why

I couldn't breathe while off the ventilator. They figured the one in my left shoulder may have been from an old PICC line; they were more concerned about the one in my lung. The doctors wanted to start me on blood thinners ASAP, but they also wanted to allow time for my lungs to heal as they were worried that thin blood would cause more bleeding.

While the doctors debated the proper dosage of blood thinner, they tried, once again, to turn down my ventilator support. Unfortunately, similar to the day before, my oxygen saturation started dropping and I started hyperventilating. They decided the best step forward was to do a tracheotomy (trach). The rationale was that since it seemed as though it was going to take a while to get me off the ventilator, the trach would help ease the transition to breathing on my own. After the trach, for which I was grateful to be knocked out, I still wasn't able to talk, but my throat felt better overall. It no longer felt as though I was constantly choking on something or swallowing glass. (When I say "trach" from here on, I'm referring to the breathing tube in my throat. The actual surgery in which they put in the tube is called a tracheotomy and the tube is called a tracheostomy, although some people, like me, use the terms interchangeably.)

When I woke up after the procedure, my family was still around so I could "chat" with them briefly. By this point, I was becoming efficient at writing everything down. I quickly learned that it was beneficial to write a summary of what a doctor or nurse said if no family member was around and make everyone read it when they came in the room. This way I didn't have to answer the same questions over and over. Even so, I killed a lot of trees during my stay in ICU.

Although my throat discomfort eased, with the trach in my anxiety returned full force. As soon as it was in, the medical team wanted me off the ventilator support as quickly as possible. I understood that they wanted my lungs to be working on their own and that it was important to start weaning off support, but it was too much, too fast. The respiratory team started "trach weaning" (that is, being off the ventilator and on supplemental oxygen) the next day. The plan was to start with a few hours off the ventilator to breathe with just the support of oxygen, slowly increasing the amount of time every day as my lungs strengthened. I had to be off the ventilator for twenty-four hours before I could be moved to the Step-Down Unit.

The problem with this plan was that my brain didn't believe that my lungs could work without oxygen, so while the RT kept telling me I would be fine, I didn't believe it. The team wasn't even trying to get me to breathe without oxygen support, but during the switch from the ventilator to oxygen I would panic. I would be without oxygen for less than a minute, but it made me anxious and I wouldn't be able to recover.

After a few incidents, I started dreading the switch and everything to do with the trach. It was a nightmare. I started to panic about being unable to get instant help if I felt I needed to go to the bathroom. The panic soon spread to whenever I felt short of breath or trapped in the bed or even at random times with no discernible trigger. This panic usually resulted in my body reacting in mysterious ways, which often meant expelling everything as quickly as possible (and you thought the poop talk was over). I did okay if I was in a chair because I could breathe easier while sitting up during the transfer, but they often wanted to do the switch-over first thing in the morning when I was still lying in bed.

I especially hated the transfer from the ventilator to oxygen when it was done by medical students. I know that students need to learn and that someone has to be their guinea pig, but I hate when it's me. The students probably had some experience with the ventilator, but one day, one of them screwed up the transfer, fumbling around with the equipment, leaving me without oxygen for seemingly forever (it was probably only a few minutes). This led to such a severe panic attack that the nurse came rushing into the room to put me back on the ventilator. It took several hours before my heart rate dropped enough for them to try the transfer again that day. After that incident, Amy talked to the RT and told her that I would be eternally grateful if I didn't have any more students work with me. The students were all friendly, but I needed to reduce my triggers and subsequent panic attacks if I was ever going to get out of intensive care. The therapist was supportive and said it wasn't a problem. From then on, she was the one to work with me, which helped reduce my stress level significantly.

I was quickly prescribed medication to help calm me down, although it never seemed to fully work. Part of the problem was that I didn't always know the triggers so I couldn't pre-medicate to avoid the panic attacks. I could only let the nurses know once I was already halfway through feeling anxious, and by the time they got the medication, I would be in full-out panic mode. The cycle was exhausting and frustrating and didn't help my recovery.

One nurse told me, in the middle of a panic attack when I didn't have medication, that I shouldn't worry about my anxiety attacks because the body can only "freak out" for about fifteen minutes at a time. All I had to do was keep telling myself that it would only be fifteen minutes of feeling like I was going to die. I didn't appreciate the advice at that moment but, surprisingly, it has helped ever since. I don't know if it's true, but even the potentially false knowledge that I can only panic, hyperventilating, for so long helps me ride it out in the moment.

The panic attacks lessened as I was moved down to less intensive care. The bed was cheaper with less cushioning, and I was getting stronger, which meant that I could haul myself into a sitting position. While I continued to panic once in a while, it was not as significant or as often. By the time I was on the regular transplant floor, the panic attacks had pretty much disappeared. At that point, I was able to get to the bathroom by myself and no longer had the trach, so both of my major triggers were gone.

I continued with physiotherapy while I was trach-weaning, which amounted to walking around the nurses' station, trying not to pass out. I had a lot of support while walking: I used a full-body walker that I just rested my arms on as I shuffled along. The physiotherapist usually held on to me while the physio assistant carried either the ventilation bag or oxygen to help me breathe. Usually, a family member walked behind me with my IV pole and a chair for when I got tired. It was always a huge ordeal to go on a little walk even though it was necessary. Some days went better than others. I was determined that I would improve quickly, but my brain was way ahead of my body on what it thought I could do.

During those days, I had one particularly frightening incident. I was walking along and kept telling the physiotherapist that I felt fine until the world suddenly started to fade away. I could hear people talking, but it was as though they were at the end of a long tunnel and everything was fuzzy. The next thing I remember is sitting in my chair with Isaiah's worried face staring at me. By writing, I asked him what had happened and he said that I zombie-walked into the room, but when they tried to get me to sit down, I refused, standing there and clenching the walker. They had to pry my hands off the walker and force me to sit in the chair. I wrote that I didn't remember anything except feeling a vague awareness of people around me. He and the physiotherapist looked concerned. Following that incident they kept checking about every minute during my walks to make sure that I was actually with them mentally.

Once I gained some strength back in my body, I started sitting up more frequently in the chair in my room. It was exhausting at first, and the most I could sit was for a few hours at a time before having to lie down again. I know it seems like such a foreign concept because most people sit for the majority of their day, but after spending days in bed, sitting was a lot of work. As my endurance gradually improved, I could sit up longer and longer. While that was positive for my body overall, it did a number on my tailbone. By the time I got out of the ICU, it was bruised and hurt all the time. I saw wound care specialists who were concerned about it, but thankfully the bruising never broke through the skin. The nurses were quite good about rotating me from side to side, but it was hard for them to get the pressure completely off my tailbone. It didn't help that I wasn't super compliant about always moving off my tailbone while sitting because I felt most comfortable in an upright position to reduce my anxiety. It was a catch-22: sit to help with my breathing and therefore reduce panic attacks or lie down and possibly panic, but relieve the pressure on my tailbone. Although neither option was particularly ideal, without consciously making the decision, minimizing my panic attacks to the detriment of my tailbone won out. It seemed there was no way for my entire body to heal at the same rate: progress with one part came at a cost for another at every point in the recovery journey.

On December 7, I was allowed to have a Popsicle. After only having dampened foam swabs and brushing my teeth as a way to rinse out my mouth, a Popsicle was a godsend. Granted, it was a gross flavour (banana!). Even so, I had never had a gross Popsicle that tasted so good. Just having something cold in my mouth felt divine. It was a joyous occasion that wasn't repeated as the doctors switched for the week (they worked weekly shifts) and the next few doctors didn't believe in the risk involved (infection and whatnot) with giving people Popsicles when they have a trach. My excitement about my progress with the Popsicle was short-lived.

The downer came soon after, when I had to go to the bathroom. The nurse got the bedpan and I went, only to have her exclaim, "Umm, this isn't good!" That is never a response one wants to hear after pooping. Instead of stool, I had basically excreted blood clots. The nurse, in what appeared to be a controlled panic, quickly left the room and called every specialist on the floor and stopped my blood thinners as well as my nasal feeds. All the residents and doctors who were around seemed to come into my room at once to inspect the blood poop. After the parade of specialists, the gastroenterology (GI) team wheeled some fancy equipment into my room and informed me that they were about to do a scope of my stomach. Due to a bad experience long ago during a stomach scope for a feeding tube, I started hyperventilating.

Thankfully, the nurse gave me a lot of knock-out medication so I don't remember anything after hearing, "We're injecting the sedation now." Turns out I had three bleeding ulcers in my stomach and upper intestine, which was why I was losing so much blood. The doctors were able to clamp them off somehow (I'm not sure how that worked exactly, but it sounded highly technical) and were sure that they had solved the problem. In the meantime, my hemoglobin had dropped significantly, so they gave me three units of blood to replace what I had lost. I had never received a blood transfusion before. I'm not sure if it was because it was my first time or because I was still high from the sedation, but I was deeply engrossed in the entire process. I learned that blood was sent up still frozen from the blood bank to the floors, which meant it was cold while going into my veins. I've had blood since, and the nurses usually let the blood thaw for a bit before infusing. But that night they seemed to put it in half-frozen. It was a strange feeling.

I bled a little the next day and showed no signs of stopping so on the ninth, the team scoped me again. They once again told me that they clamped off the ulcer that was still bleeding. The doctor kept referring to it as a "super ulcer," which was unnerving as I thought an ICU GI doctor would see ulcers all the time. It wasn't terribly comforting when he would make comments like, "You have a super ulcer!", "We got the super ulcer!", or, "Where did this super ulcer come from?" The doctor sounded as if he had respect for my super ulcer and wanted to study it further. No one could tell me the cause of the ulcers and just chalked them up as a "thing that happens sometimes." It could have been caused by my blood thinners, the overall stress on my body, various medications, or all of those combined.

While all the doctors were hanging out in my room, they pulled out the last two of my chest tubes. It's hard to describe how chest tubes feel other than being a pressure on the body and lungs. Because I had them all inserted during the transplant, it was hard to know what pressure was from the tubes and what was from the incision. Having the tubes pulled out didn't exactly hurt (except when the doctor nicked my skin while removing the stitches) but created a weird pressure that was built up and then suddenly released. One of the tubes was stitched in a way that hurt when I tried to roll on that side, so it was a relief to have it gone. Overall, it felt like a good step forward to have two more lines out.

After the ulcers and internal bleeding, the GI doctors and transplant doctors had a hard time deciding if they should leave me on the blood thinners. The GI doctor wanted them to stop because he felt that I might still be bleeding slightly from the ulcers, while the transplant doctor wanted me to stay on them to try and break up the blood clot in my lung. Eventually, the transplant doctor won the day, but they watched me closely.

1 2

ICU TIME

By this time, you may be wondering how one stays clean while lying in a hospital bed for weeks on end. The answer is, frankly, you don't. The nurses would sometimes do a "sponge bath" of sorts, which involved wiping me down with pre-soaped cloths. They were warmish, which I think was supposed to help me feel clean but just made me sticky. It was not ideal. My hair was also a mess. I had kept it short thinking that it would be easier to look after while I was in the hospital. In retrospect, it worked fine because I wore a headband every day, but it may have been easier if it had been longer so I could have thrown it in a ponytail.

Immediately post-transplant, the nurses didn't like to wash my hair because of the risk of getting water on any of the fancy equipment or down the ETT. They used shower caps instead. The idea is that they put the shower cap on, shake up the hair, leave it on for five minutes, comb out the hair, and presto: all clean. They don't work; they just caused a massive dandruff rain. The no-rinse shampoo in the cap is great theoretically and may have worked if the quality of the shampoo had been better, but as the hospital didn't have the budget for more than one-ply toilet paper, they weren't about to spring for Lush dry shampoo.

Occasionally, if the nurses weren't busy, there were a few of them who would wash my hair with real shampoo and water. It doesn't seem like much, but little things like clean hair helped to keep my mood elevated during my long stay. I felt better after every hair wash. Once I was able to sit in a chair, my family could awkwardly wash my hair with basins, but it was always a hassle

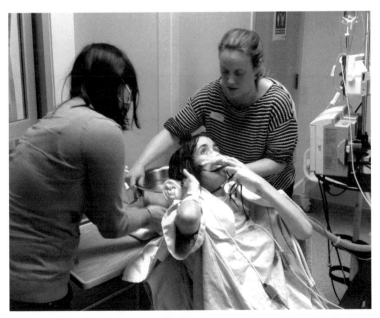

Two friends wash Allison's hair at the Toronto General Hospital in 2014, shortly after her transplant. Little things like clean hair helped elevate Allison's mood during her long stay. (Isaiah Jacques)

so I didn't like to harass them to do it often. Eventually in the Step-Down Unit, there were care workers who did daily sponge baths with actual water which felt glorious. I quickly got over the "naked in front of strangers" shyness because it was either that or never be clean. There wasn't much of an option.

***

After the chest drainage tubes were removed, my daily chest x-ray showed I had some minor fluid buildup in my lungs. On December 14, I was scheduled for a CT scan to determine if there was enough to warrant putting the tubes back in. Instead of heading down for the scan, I pooped out "a lake of blood," as the nurse exclaimed. It was not a good start to the day, especially for my nurse who had to deal with it at the beginning of her shift (welcome to work!). My hemoglobin levels were crazy low, so once again my nurse rightfully panicked and summoned the doctors.

The doctors did yet another GI scope that I was sedated for, which showed a small bleed from my super ulcer. The one upside was that there was a small clot around it, showing that my body was at least trying to heal itself. Unfortunately, it was not enough to completely stop the bleeding so they added yet another clip (I don't know what these clips are made of or how they work), added more "please behave" spray to my stomach, and took a biopsy to see if I had a random "let's grow ulcers" bacteria in my stomach. Fortunately, I didn't and the ulcers calmed down after that final scope.

When I woke up, I was quite hungry and thirsty because they had stopped my feeds at the first sign of bleeding. The floor manager had also switched my room and the food services staff didn't have the updated information, so they kept delivering food to my room all day. In my hunger and thirst, I wanted to down the cartons of milk and juice before the nurse noticed, except the problem would then be that I would aspirate and die; it was best that I restrain myself. I was still desperate for ice chips or water, anything to ease the incessant cotton-mouth. The Popsicle was a distant memory at this point. When I brushed my teeth, the nurses were adamant that I spit out the water I used to rinse my mouth, while I was always tempted to swallow it just because it would've made my throat feel so much better. I didn't, of course, as I was paranoid about aspirating and didn't want to die from toothpaste water after going through so much. My nurse restarted the feeds slowly, after getting the okay from the doctor. I think she was tired of me complaining every time she came to check on me.

I was determined December 15 would be the day I finally managed to trach mask for twenty-four hours. I had been off the ventilator since 6:30 A.M. and was determined to go for twenty-four hours—that was all I needed to get out of the ICU and into the Step-Down Unit. It was honestly all I could think about. My life revolved around that trach and whether or not I could last twenty-four hours without the ventilator. I was doing fairly well; I felt good and anxiety-free until the afternoon.

That afternoon on the floor was pure chaos. Absolute pandemonium. Thankfully, it had very little to do with me, for once, and Mom and I were able to sit and watch the drama. One minute after my nurse went on break, the charge nurse burst into my room and announced that I was to be moved "temporarily" to a new floor. Right that second! They needed my room because someone with greater priority was moving in.

The nurse who was covering the shift mentioned that since I was already sitting up, I should be transported to the new floor in a wheelchair. I wrote that that sounded like a good idea, which soon became, "The patient demands that she be transported down in a wheelchair." While they scrambled to find a chair for me, I kept trying to sign that I was honestly okay with being transferred back to bed for the ride. I thought I was being asked which one I preferred, I wasn't demanding anything. The porter (*transport*, as they were known there) brought up a wheelchair for me and had me all ready to go.

At that moment, my nurse sauntered in, late from her break, complaining that the elevators were crammed by people rushing down to the basement for the free hot chocolate being given out to staff. Already slightly high-strung, she did not react well to the news that she was being shipped off to a new floor and started demanding answers as to why she had to be the one to move. She tried to refuse and fought with the charge nurse outside my room, so it was another thirty minutes before anything happened while I sat there with the transport.

After much more debate about how the equipment would be moved, I was transferred back to my bed and whisked off to, I think, the Acute Post-Op Area (still not sure if that's where I was) for the night. It was a giant open ward where people hung out after surgery. It was not conducive to one-to-one nursing or anything relaxing. There were three patients, including me, kicked out of their rooms that night for the new influx of transplant ICU patients. The man beside me was rather medically out of it, but he still kept trying to pull out his trach and other lines. The nurses had to repeatedly ask that he not pull out the lines, which got tiresome to hear.

As expected when people are suddenly whisked to new locations in hospital, nothing was prepared for the nurses or patients. The nurses had to set up their new medication system and gather supplies from various floors. Everyone kept running back and forth between floors while complaining and swearing about how unfortunate their lives were. They also had to figure out the different equipment like "how to use the thermometer" from the new floor. It was not the environment I had envisioned when I set out to complete my twenty-four-hour trach-weaning attempt.

There was nowhere for Mom and Isaiah to sit because the ward wasn't designed for visitors either. They found terrible plastic chairs from somewhere but they weren't comfortable. Everything was in an open area so they didn't stay long. My nurse was sitting more or less at the end of my bed, and I could see all the other patients around me. By evening, the novelty of being in a new place was over when the RT was the one from that floor instead of the one I was used to. I was starting to feel extremely anxious around 11:00 P.M., but there were no anti-anxiety medications brought down for me. A nurse had to go back to the ICU department to get my medication but decided that he would go on break and "bring the medication down after." That's fine when it's a routine issue but doesn't work when breathing seems at stake.

It all went downhill after that. I couldn't bring myself down from my panic attack. I got myself more and more worked up so that eventually the nurse had to call in the RT to put me back on the ventilator. Much to their surprise, the day RT had only wheeled down the ventilation machine and hadn't set anything up. The nurse had to bag me for a solid five minutes while the night shift RT tried to set up the machine.

Once my oxygen saturation returned to normal, I felt better while being bagged. Because I'm stubborn and refuse to say no, I agreed to try the trach mask again. I thought maybe since I had calmed down from the attack, I would do okay. Nope! Another round of panicking occurred and back on the bag I went while the RT figured out what was happening with the machine. Mercifully, almost five minutes back on the ventilator and with my medication finally arriving, I went to sleep and slept soundly until 6:30 A.M.

The next day was much less crazy as the nurses had settled into their new spots and all the supplies had finally made it down to the new floor. I, however, woke up annoyed that I hadn't made it twenty-four hours without the ventilator. I was frustrated because my oxygen saturation had been fine but all my hopes had been thwarted by a mental response. I had tried listening to music and doing all the counting exercises that people had recommended, but nothing worked until I got the medication and was back on the ventilator.

I started again that morning, determined to make it twenty-four hours off the ventilator. My nurse (again the high-strung one) washed my hair, which was simply magnificent; I think she was bored in this new unit. During the hair-washing, my nurse got the call that we were moving back up to ICU. I was transferred back into the bed, everything was piled around me, and I immediately began to panic. Unlike last time when I was able to watch the entire move with amusement, I had another anxiety attack about being back in bed.

This time, my nurse had one dose of medication ready for me and talked me through most of it. I got a second dose when someone else was brought down to the floor to assist in the move. The rest of the dose, plus time, seemed to help bring me back to myself. All the nurses kept reminding me that it was normal to have panic attacks while being in ICU. They claimed that almost everyone has one at some point and that most of the ICU population is on some type of anti-anxiety medication. The fact that it's normal did not make it any less scary when it happened.

Upon my return to ICU, I was put in a different room than the one I had left. This time I had a roommate, which I wasn't expecting, but since he was on dialysis and waiting for a kidney, he was relatively quiet. His mother, who constantly prayed over him, was the one who made more noise. Roommates and their families are annoying. The positive part of being in the new room was that my bed faced a window, and I saw sunshine for the first time in twenty-three days. There was a pretty sunset that evening, which made the craziness from the previous two days more bearable.

I love sunsets, so much so that I've been known to drag my family out at dusk to find the perfect vantage point for watching one. Other than freezing on cliffs in Newfoundland, the only time this was a problem was when Amy and I were travelling in Italy in 2007. Amy wanted to spend the afternoon in a Tuscan town, and I wanted to see a sunset over the Tuscan landscape. We booked a shared room at a hostel in Florence, packed a day bag, and hopped on a train heading out of the city to a town recommended in our guidebook. After about twenty minutes and three stops on what was supposed to be a fifteen-minute train ride, we realized we did not recognize any of the towns that were being announced. We had a sinking sensation that we were on the wrong train. Since we didn't know where the train was headed, we jumped off at the next stop, believing this town would be just as beautiful as our original destination. We were disappointed: it was a cute town with delicious fresh cherries and rabbits hopping around the local park, but after an hour we had exhausted every activity. I convinced Amy we should get on the next train to travel to the next town in hope it would have a beautiful sunset.

The train arrived before we had given much consideration to our decision. Ten minutes later, it passed through a tunnel in a mountain, and we finally realized how late it was getting. We decided it was time to abandon our plan and head back to Florence. We got off at the next stop, consulted the schedule posted on the side of the tiny train station, and were relieved to read that there was one more train heading back to Florence in an hour. So we waited, ate more cherries, and hoped the train would be early.

The hour came and went. That was when we started to panic. We double- and triple-checked the schedule, but since we couldn't read Italian, we could only look at the times and wonder why the train hadn't arrived. There was an asterisk beside the train time, but we couldn't decipher what it signified. It was dark by this point, so we left the station (which was basically a small wooden shelter), only to realize it was outside of the actual town. There were no houses around, and the only thing we could see was a graveyard across the street. We figured it was best to stay at the tiny station. Regretfully, we resigned ourselves to spending a long, cold night there. At this point I was profusely apologizing to Amy who looked like she might murder someone at the mention of sunset. My quips about our cherries warding off starvation were also not appreciated.

As we were figuring out which of the two wooden benches looked the most comfortable, a man arrived speaking rapid Italian, punctuated by energetic hand gestures. We gestured that we had been waiting for the train and didn't know what to do. He sighed and said in broken English that the train we were waiting for only ran on weekends, or maybe he said it never ran on weekends. We never did figure that out. Either way, there was no train coming to take us back to Florence. He motioned for us to follow him, and I quickly checked the next day's schedule before leaving. The first train would be at 6:40 A.M.; I resolved then that we would be on it.

The man took us to what seemed to be the town hall where people were playing cards and drinking. Everyone proceeded to have a loud, lengthy discussion with a lot of hand-waving and gesturing in our direction while we stood in the corner. Eventually, a cellphone was thrust into Amy's hand, and the British man on the other end of the line explained that the man who had handed her the phone was going to take us to a house where we could spend the night. Amy asked him if we could pay for someone to drive us back to Florence instead. He replied "No, it would cost too much and no one wants to drive at this hour." It seemed we had no choice, so we followed the woman chosen to be the one to take in the crazy Canadians.

Her home was a few streets down from the town hall and we were introduced to her family, who were also playing cards and smoking. Fortunately, we had a puffer with us which we both used before tucking into the large, comfortable bed they offered us to sleep in. It was much nicer than the single beds waiting back at the hostel. Having agreed to try to catch the 6:40 A.M. train, we rose early and quietly snuck out of the house.

Back at the train station, we waited for the train. When it didn't arrive, we cursed, double- and triple-checked the train schedule—again—and finally noticed that "6h40" also had an asterisk beside it. This could have meant anything, but at any rate, the train wasn't arriving. The next train was only an hour and a half later. We had never been so happy to see a locomotive in our lives.

When we finally returned to Florence, the man who ran the hostel said he had waited up for us. We apologized, tried with little success to explain what had happened, and crept to our room to do our aerosol masks and get ready for our day of sightseeing. The ironic part about the entire experience was that later that night when we sat at the top of a Florentine hill eating more fresh cherries, we watched the most beautiful sunset over the Tuscan hillside. Sometimes, it's good to simply appreciate where you are.

From the hospital room with a window, I enjoyed watching the first sunset I had seen in more than three weeks. The next day I finally got my catheter out; another line gone! It was a big step to be told that I could pee on my own. That day I was finally successful at making it twenty-four hours off the ventilator and breathing without equipment (though with oxygen). It was a huge step.

I needed medication to make it through, but make it through I did. I still needed one major suctioning during the day because I had trouble coughing up the junk in my lungs. That concerned one of the doctors, but since I made it through without a full-blown panic attack and stayed off the machine, the RT took the ventilator out of my room. I was finally making steps to get out of the ICU before Christmas. I was given some orange juice to swab my mouth, which was a flavour explosion to my tongue. I was longing for food and water like they were going out of style.

The next day, after forty-eight hours of being off the ventilator, the doctors switched my tracheotomy to a smaller one. It happened so fast that I didn't even have time to be nervous or get anxious. Two of the respiratory doctors came in to see how I was doing. I indicated that I was proud to finally be off the ventilator and asked if that meant that my trach could be removed. They were not a fan of the idea because I still couldn't cough up the crap in my lungs and required occasional suctioning. They did, however, agree that it could be downgraded to a smaller one, which would help my throat heal faster. With that, they consulted the computer (it looked to me as though they were reading instructions), found the right size trach, put on gloves, and gave medication to help me relax. It felt as if one resident yanked out the trach while the other one shoved the new one in my throat. I had a panic attack as soon as they left, though, and Mom, who had watched the entire procedure from the visitor's chair, went off to find a nurse to get me more medication.

A nurse came in shortly after I had calmed down to announce that since I was no longer on the ventilator, I was being transferred to the Step-Down Unit. Now. Once a decision is made, everything happens rather quickly.

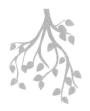

1 3

STEPS FORWARD
IN STEP-DOWN

On December 20, after three and a half weeks in ICU, I finally made it down the hallway to transplant Step-Down. I was quite proud that I was able to walk over to the Step-Down Unit, with help from the physiotherapist. One of the nurses joked that it was showing off, but after three and a half weeks in ICU, I was anxious to get out of there. Step-Down is considered a different unit even though it's on the same floor, just in a different corner of the hallway. I was still connected to the heart monitor and blood pressure, heart rate, and oxygen saturation machines. The only tangible differences were that the nursing staff was at a two-to-one ratio, the beds were less expensive, and they gave the patients call bells. I had a private room with a glass window through which I could stare at my nurse, so other than the different bed and slightly less intensive nursing care, it wasn't much different.

The less expensive beds served me well during my now infrequent panic attacks because the firmness meant I could haul myself into a sitting position more easily. It was not as good for my tailbone though, which was still hurting. The physiotherapist on Step-Down gave me a gel cushion to put on my chair, which relieved some of the pressure while I was sitting. There wasn't much more they could do other than tell me to shift positions every fifteen to twenty minutes and try to stand up as much as possible (which still wasn't often as my legs were weak).

The other change on the floor was a new set of nurses, a new physiotherapist, and different RT. I was already acquainted with the physiotherapist from the outpatient clinic because he occasionally covered shifts while I was pre-transplant; it was nice to see a familiar face. The RTs for Step-Down didn't seem to work regular shifts, so I never got to know any of them as well as the ones on ICU.

Once I was settled into the Step-Down Unit, the doctor said that I was allowed ice chips as long as I promised to eat about "ten ice chips an hour." It was more of a "you can have ice chips if you promise not to shove the entire cup in your mouth at once" caution. I promised to not overindulge and I was given the precious ice chips. Ice had never tasted so good. Ever since the one night where I was allowed a Popsicle, I had dreamed about being able to drink something. It was heavenly. I'm not sure that anyone who has been without real water for more than twenty days can truly understand. Let's just say that I hope you're never in that situation, but if you are, you'll know how wonderful it feels to be allowed to have liquids again.

Since I still had some fluid in my lungs, on what seemed to be a Hail Mary effort on the part of the transplant doctors to get rid of it without putting the chest tubes back in, they increased the dosage of my diuretic, or pee-like-a-racehorse medication. Since it dries out everything, I was extra thankful to have ice chips. I peed all night long, and by the next day, the Winter Solstice, I was informed that the medication had worked! The daily x-ray showed that the fluid was draining well, so the doctors decided against reinserting the chest tubes. It took a lot of stress off me to hear that I wouldn't need more chest tubes, even though the team had repeatedly told me it was normal for them to sometimes be reinserted. Every time some sort of setback happened, the team always told me that was "normal," although the Almighty Transplant Manual hadn't mentioned anything about ulcers or clots.

The big step of that day was that I could start talking! I still had the trach but since I had moved to the smaller size and was no longer on the ventilator, the RT decided it was time to move to the next step. She put a plastic stopper called a "cork" (maybe it used to be made of cork) over the hole in the trach and then I could breathe normally. The process is called "corking," and I needed to be corked for forty-eight hours to move to the seventh floor. When the cork was in, the airflow no longer went out my throat, which meant I could talk. Well, in fact, I could whisper slightly while squeaking loudly every so often like an adolescent boy. I hadn't realized how hard it would be to talk again and how much my throat muscles would deteriorate after the transplant. My poor vocal cords were in shock from suddenly being in demand. Otherwise, I felt comfortable while corking. I was still on oxygen via nasal prongs, which I didn't really need but it was there as a security blanket. When the RT had tried taking me off the oxygen completely, my saturations stayed level, but I started panicking.

My brain was not ready to admit that my lungs could handle room air. Stupid brain, panicking about everything. Silly brain, our lungs *worked*!

When Mom came in that day—her last day of visiting before heading back to New Brunswick—she almost burst into tears when I managed to croak out a squeaky hello. The RT forbade me from writing anything down as she wanted me to focus on strengthening my vocal cords now, but I found I still had to dig out the pen and paper when I got tired. My voice was so weak that it was hard for people to understand what I was saying. This meant repeating sentences often, which was tiring.

Things held steady for a few days. The diuretic worked well, drying out my lungs and reducing the swelling in my elephant feet. I was finally allowed to go without compression stockings which was a reprieve for my dried-out legs. Although I went through loads of moisturizer during my hospital stay, I felt like I never could catch up with the effects of the dry air.

Since I was doing well with the corking and my voice was slowly getting stronger, the nurses, tired of me always asking for more water, called in the speech language pathologist (SLP). I had never considered that the muscles in the throat would deteriorate as fast as leg muscles, but because they often do, the SLP has to do a swallow assessment before patients are allowed liquids or solid foods after a transplant. The swallow assessment consisted of analyzing tongue and throat strength, chewing ice chips, and swallowing a few teaspoons of water. I did well enough on the assessment that I was allowed twelve sips of water an hour on top of my occasional ice chips.

I realize that doesn't sound like anything, but it was so satisfying. To be honest, when the speech pathologist had me swallow the first teaspoon of water, I thought I was going to sink into the floor out of sheer contentment. I sucked back my water allotment all day, happily.

The hardest part about not being able to eat or drink was seeing the nurses walk around with their Starbucks coffee cups. They would sit on the other side of the partition and sip away while I sat in bed so thirsty. It was like a weird form of torture. I mentioned it to one nurse and she said that it was just regular tea but since I didn't know what they were drinking, I dreamed of caramel and frothy chai lattes. The longer I went without food or liquids, the more I dreamed of everything I was missing.

Part two of the swallow assessment, a videofluoroscopic swallowing study, came the next day. I was excited to have this done because I was anxious to start getting different types of food. Since it was around the holidays, I had been told the SLP may not be able to squeeze me in before the Christmas break. That would've meant at least another three days of nothing but water. I was determined to start eating food again; the liquid diet through my nasal tube was not filling me anymore, and I was frequently hungry.

For the assessment, I was taken down to a small room where I was placed behind an x-ray machine and was fed different types of thickened liquids and soft foods. The food was laced with barium so the SLP could watch in real time how the food went down my throat. She wanted to make sure nothing was going into my trach and that my epiglottis was working after about a month of not doing anything.

I had a minor panic attack while in the room and started shaking out of cold and fear. The SLP didn't want to give me any anti-anxiety medication as she said that would relax my muscles too much and make the test even harder. I think I had put so much pressure on myself to get it right that I was panicked about failing and imagined not being able to eat or drink anything for weeks.

The SLP started out with thickened water which sounds gross, and would be under any other circumstance, but to me was delicious. At that point, anything that would help my dry mouth was welcome. She followed that up with thickened juice, soft bread, Jell-O, and digestive cookies. Under normal conditions, I would absolutely despise these soggy foods; however, after not eating anything for almost a month, they were the best things I had ever consumed. The SLP would put the liquid or soft food in my mouth and I would hold it there for a few seconds before being prompted to swallow. The first few times were rough, but eventually I figured out how to slow down (not panic) and simply focus on what I was doing. I especially slowed down when she started putting the soft food in my mouth. The apple juice and applesauce were easy to eat slowly as they tasted so good, even with the barium.

All went down once I managed to relax, but it did take me several swallows to get down the stickier foods like the mashed potatoes. Thankfully, I didn't aspirate on anything. In the end I was allowed to have soft foods and thickened liquids. It was exactly what I expected after almost choking on the spoonful of potatoes. There was a list of guidelines for me to follow, which I only half-listened to because I was so excited about the idea of a smoothie. The SLP said I had to use a spoon for all the thickened liquids, no straws; that I shouldn't try to chug anything (as if that was something I could even do); focus whenever I was swallowing; and to try to swallow three times for every spoonful. There were many instructions to ensure that I got all the food down so nothing got stuck. I was also told to finish every meal with some water to ensure that there was nothing stuck on the trach.

As soon as the SLP said I was allowed smoothies, Isaiah's sisters (who were visiting over Christmas) rushed down to Booster Juice to get me one. They returned with my Christmas smoothie (it was the twenty-third after all). It was everything I had been dreaming about for the last three weeks. Due to the

SLP's instructions to "swallow intentionally" and "three swallows for each spoonful," I only made it through half of the beverage before it melted so much that it was probably no longer considered a "thick liquid." Isaiah had to finish it for me.

With the arrival of supper, my excitement about being allowed food came crashing down. I quickly realized how hard it was to swallow actual food. It was astonishing how good it tasted, but I was exhausted after a few small bites of applesauce and mashed potatoes. I felt discouraged because I had managed only about four regular bites of food; the dietitian wouldn't remove my nasal tube until I was eating full meals. The road to get to that point seemed awfully long.

⚜

I've always had a weird relationship with food. Children with CF are often malnourished due to their inability to absorb nutrients from food, and I was no different. Digestive enzymes are required to help break down food, and even using them, there is often a struggle to gain or maintain weight. When I was a toddler, a lot of the time I would refuse to eat or eat and throw up afterward. I didn't do this on purpose; my stomach simply didn't want to keep food down. It was concerning for everyone because I was quickly becoming malnourished. I simply wasn't able to absorb all the nutrients I needed from the small amount of food I ate. The doctors initially told my parents it was a power play and that I wasn't eating in order to gain control of them. I'm not sure why they thought a one-year-old would throw up food as a method of control. My patient parents tried bribing me with stickers to eat my food, then giving me time-outs when I still wouldn't eat, then back to the stickers. The doctors inserted a "temporary" feeding tube to bypass my stomach and give my body a chance to gain weight. It helped immensely. I started putting weight on, but still wouldn't eat much orally.

The doctors were able to accurately diagnose my eating problems only when my parents hospitalized me at the IWK for three weeks while they visited Australia. The hospitalization was on the advice of one of the Halifax CF doctors who was a big believer in self-care (and if anyone needed a break, it was my parents, who were raising a ten-month-old, a three-year-old with CF who wouldn't eat, and a seven-year-old with CF). Amy stayed with family friends and David went to our grandparents' house. I was hospitalized so Mom and Dad wouldn't have to worry about teaching someone to do my tubal feeds for three weeks. Since I was in the hospital already, the doctors sent me to a psychologist who figured out my brain was simply not telling me to eat. I don't remember this time at the hospital so it clearly wasn't traumatizing. I'm told another family "adopted" me, and my relatives who lived nearby visited often. My feeding tube remained until I was around seven, when I was eating enough orally to gain weight without the supplementation.

Once I was eating food regularly as a kid, I was possibly the pickiest eater in Canada. I would refuse to eat anything that had a garnish or lumpy texture. I would live on biscuits and jam for a month before deciding I never wanted to eat another biscuit again. Mom would try to sneak all the calories she could into various meals. The desserts she made for Amy and me were always high-calorie and high-fat. We went through a phase of eating peanut butter pie every week until we both reached the point where we never wanted to see peanut butter again. David probably has weird issues with food too because all the junk food in the house was "for his sisters," so maybe he shouldn't eat all the cookies. It was fortunate that he was such an active kid with good metabolism, or he might have gained a lot of weight growing up in our household.

As a result of my struggle to gain weight, I have an unusual relationship with food compared to most people. My entire pre-transplant life, I had been told by dietitians that I needed to focus on either maintaining or gaining weight with a daily diet of 2,500 to 3,000 calories. As a result, I have a skewed view of healthy eating and guilt associated with food. Most people feel guilty when they eat a piece of cake; I feel guilty if I don't eat the piece of cake. Unlike most people, I need to buy the option with the highest calories at the grocery store and make sure I don't fill up on lettuce before getting to the main meal to ensure that I maximize my calorie intake.

I've become a much better eater as an adult. Now I think I have a normal level of pickiness, although I still avoid oddly textured foods like Jell-O and celery because, well, they're gross. Staying with other families in my travels and politely eating what they've made for me forced me to eat a lot of foods I thought were terrible. But it turns out whipped cream is delicious. Who knew?

Because of this struggle to gain weight, I've always been slim. As an adult, I've had strangers helpfully tell me to eat a hamburger. I'm not sure why people think it appropriate to comment on a random woman's weight. The usual response when I mentioned needing to gain weight was, "I can give you some of mine," or, "I wish I had that problem." I brushed it off, and people usually stopped offering advice once I talked about having to supplement my diet with Boost and Ensure. I know that most people struggle with wanting to lose weight so when I frame it as a weight issue, instead of an "I get to eat whatever I want" situation, people tend to be more sympathetic and give me fewer angry glares when I eat a chocolate bar in front of them.

In the weeks following my transplant, the struggle to eat again was an aspect of the post-surgery that had never crossed my mind. I knew I would be fed through a nasal tube during the transplant process, but I never imagined that it would be hard to resume eating. I had not considered my throat and esophagus as muscles and that, just like my vocal cords, they would shrink from lack of use. The transplant manual could've mentioned something helpful like, "Every single muscle in your body will shrink and need to be rebuilt, even the ones you have never considered before; be prepared to learn how to eat again!"

Since I was eating a little, the nurses decided that I should try swallowing my pills. I refused at first because it was exhausting to eat thickened juice, let alone try to swallow a crushed pill. I thought I should spend my energy on food textures other than applesauce. While some of them gave me a bit of a hard time, they all said it was okay for a few days but added, "You need to try soon!" It wasn't that I didn't want to try; it was more that I didn't have the energy. I wasn't being defiant without reason.

Growing up, I generally never had a problem swallowing pills. Mom and Dad had powder digestive enzymes that they mixed in applesauce when Amy and I were too small to swallow pills, but it didn't take long for us to adjust to the capsules. There was some competition between Amy and me: if she could swallow all eight of her supper pills at once, so could I. It also made sense to swallow as many as possible in one go so as not to fill up on liquid before the meal. Somehow our brother, David, missed the "pill swallowing gene" and would struggle any time he had to take a pill. Amy and I would mock him endlessly, which probably didn't help, while Mom would have to mix them, crushed, into yogurt, or later, hide the medication in a nutty chocolate bar. Thankfully, David didn't need medication often. (I'm told he is much better about swallowing pills now.)

So the nurses continued to shoot pills up my nose, well, through my nasal tube. I think they were all pushing for me to take my own pills so that they wouldn't have to mix and crush them. All my medication—anti-rejection pills, antibiotics, and vitamins—were ground up, mixed with saline, put into a giant syringe, and shot through the tube. My digestive enzymes were mixed with the liquid feeds. If I was trying to eat something on my own, the nurse would occasionally put a digestive enzyme through the tube. To be honest though, I ate so little that I doubt my body was struggling to digest the two bites of mashed potatoes I managed to swallow.

It took longer than I would have liked, but eventually I was able to eat normally again. Since the transplant, being on a steroid all the time has increased my appetite enough that I'm finally at a healthy weight. Visits with the CF dietitian are no longer all about how to sneak extra calories into my day, and I'm off the extra meal replacements to maintain my weight. It's remarkably refreshing not to have to worry about calories for the first time in my life.

14

CHRISTMAS IN THE HOSPITAL

Christmas has always been a fun holiday in my family. We try to keep the presents to a minimum but go all out with the meals. We usually spend Christmas Eve day doing meal prep, and once that's done and much food has been consumed for dinner, we spend the evening filling each other's stockings. It's a tradition our family has observed since we never had a "Santa." As children we would fill the stockings of the adults with presents and stuff the empty space with fruit or kitchenware. Sometimes we would fill stockings with figurines taken from the manger scene—the weirder the better. As adults, we fill the stockings of our siblings, and it often gets out of hand. On Christmas Day, we would open our stockings and have a large meal with all the extended family. It's family time that I have always cherished.

The Christmas while I was waiting for the transplant was quiet with just Isaiah and me. We filled up each other's stockings and Skyped with family at home. David and Cindy flew in that night so we did have family around to celebrate with, which was enjoyable.

Christmas Day in the hospital post-transplant was similar to any other hospital day, except for seeing the slew of visitors from Isaiah's family, spending time on Skype with my family at home, and generally feeling overrun by everything around me. To start off, the RT working that day decided it would be a great Christmas present to me if he removed my trach. It was supposed to be taken out around 11:30 A.M., so while part of me was excited at the idea, the other part decided it would be fun to have a panic attack at 11:15 A.M. All it took at that point to set off a panic attack was to be told that I was having a new procedure. I told the therapist to ignore my panicking and pull it out. He didn't think that was a good idea because my oxygen saturation was dropping, and I kept getting more and more worked up imagining the trach being wrenched out of my throat. He said he would return in the afternoon to try again.

Shortly after he left, Isaiah's family showed up with a massive number of presents, and I was quickly fatigued. Although my coordination had greatly improved, I was still having problems focusing on more than one thing for long periods of time. I found it hard to concentrate on anything at all when there were so many people chatting around me and wrapping paper was flying everywhere. I ended up kicking everyone out and felt bad about it until I had a refreshing nap. Isaiah brought in a few presents a day for the next week so I wouldn't be as flooded by so many at once. It was not an exciting Christmas.

Since I was napping when he returned, the therapist decided that maybe the next day would be better to remove the trach. I felt as though I had failed. Even though I knew that anxiety attacks were normal and that it was ridiculous to feel as though I had let myself down, I couldn't help but be disappointed. I was annoyed that something that was supposed to be routine ended up being a source of anxiety for me, yet learning that I had a clot or an ulcer didn't elicit the same reaction. I'm thankful that my anxiety attacks were acute because I can't imagine having to deal with anxiety on a daily basis. I have great respect for anyone who experiences anxiety regularly. It must be so hard just to get through the day.

On Boxing Day, with the help of one RT, a nurse, two anti-anxiety pills, and lots of mantra self-chanting of, "I can do this, don't panic, I can do this, don't panic...," the trach finally came out. As I had been told—but didn't believe—it wasn't a big procedure. It felt weird but wasn't painful. The RT literally pulled the trach out of my throat and stuck a large bandage over the site. The nurse was not happy with his handiwork so she fixed it with a proper bandage. As long as the bandage was airtight, I could talk, but as soon as the seal was broken even slightly, I could only make ghost-like noises because the air would come out the hole in my throat instead of my mouth. (It didn't take long for the hole to heal over enough so that I could talk again, but until it reached that point, I had to cover the hole with my finger in order to get any noise out.)

Isaiah showed up seconds after the trach was removed, which was the perfect distraction for my anxiety. We tried to go for a short walk (I had finally been cleared go with family), but my stats dropped too much before we had gone even one step. I think it was all the medication, lack of sleep, and anxiety. Instead, we half-heartedly played cards, which turned into Isaiah reading to me, which turned into a day-long nap for me.

The trach was finally out, I was breathing on my own (with some oxygen), and I had one less thing to worry about.

It turned out that having the trach removed wasn't as transformative as I had been hoping. My throat was raw, and while I had been drinking smoothies and sips of water as often as possible, nothing was making it feel better. That night I slept well for the first half of the evening, thanks to my sleeping pills, only to wake up feeling like there was something tickling in my lungs and I needed to cough. Under normal circumstances, when I feel this sensation, I just cough a few times and it goes away. The problem now was that I still didn't have any muscle tone for coughing. Nevertheless, I kept trying to clear the tickle through my feeble coughing because I thought that whatever was bothering my lungs would soon affect my breathing. The nurse, realizing I was awake and struggling, came in and assured me that my oxygen saturation was fine, it wasn't something necessary to focus on, try to sleep, etc. It was too little, too late. Suddenly, all I could think about was getting rid of the rattle in my lungs.

If I had still had the trach in, I could've coughed until the phlegm moved to the upper airways and the nurse would've suctioned it out, but since the trach was gone, suctioning wasn't an option. I was determined to cough it out myself. Unfortunately, I totally exhausted myself trying, which then decreased my oxygen saturations, which made me panic more. I am an expert at self-fulling prophecies.

The nurse called in the RT, who seemed annoyed at being called at 3:00 A.M. The RT initially tried to suction out the mucous through my nose but failed because I panicked when the tubing hit the back of my throat. She then tried to suction through the hole in my throat. That attempt cleared my lungs somewhat but not as well as she would've liked. She tried to put the trach back in as she muttered that it had been removed too early, but it didn't work. Although the hole hadn't completely healed over, it had healed enough so that she couldn't get it in.

Eventually, she just cranked up my oxygen, re-suctioned through the hole in my throat, and lectured me on how I needed to learn to cough (as if I didn't already know). She left a strongly worded note for the doctors recommending that they put the trach back in during my one-month post-transplant bronchoscopy that was scheduled for the next day. The entire process took place over the span of an hour: a long, horrible hour. I crashed out after she left, exhausted, traumatized, and emotionally drained.

The next morning, I had my bronch. The doctors did it in my room and as far as bronchs go, it was easy. I was completely knocked out after swallowing the freezing spray, and I only woke up once they were clearing the equipment out of the room. My first question was to ask in a panic if they had put the trach back in only to fall back asleep before I heard the answer. However, since I could ask questions, it meant they had not put it back in, which was great news to me. I woke up again when the doctor returned to explain to me how much they had suctioned out of my lungs, but I fell back asleep during his explanation. I'm not sure why doctors think they can explain anything to patients who they've just pumped full of sedation.

Whatever they had sucked out of my lungs changed the feeling of my lungs and breathing. It finally felt as though everything was one organ and I no longer had to make an extra effort to breathe through different lobes. The best description I have of how my lungs felt before was that when someone asked me to breathe deeply, it took me several seconds because I had to activate each lobe separately. Suddenly, everything was working in synch. It all made sense now, why no one could tell me what it was like to breathe with separate lobes: because that's not how people normally breathe. Everything had finally clicked together, and it felt sensational.

15

THE WOUND
FROM HELL

My lungs were finally working well when I suddenly had a new problem. My incision site from the transplant had been oozing for about a week before the bronchoscopy. No one thought it was a problem because the discharge was clear. Since I was on the "make you pee" medication at the time, the nurses assumed it was normal drainage, that is, until it was time to remove half of the staples along the incision site (yes, I was stapled together). The doctor who removed the staples thought the discharge looked concerning so he swabbed the area to make sure that it wasn't an infection.

In the interim, he started me on an antibiotic as a precautionary measure.

During the bronchoscopy, the doctors opened up part of the incision where it had been oozing and cleaned out the drainage gunk. The team was worried by the amount that came out, so they scheduled a CT scan to see if the infection—if it was an infection—was anywhere else. I was also referred to the wound care nurse to get a consult on the best way to treat it. That's when I met a person who loved her job more than anything else in the world. The wound care nurse was so excited to see me and my wound. She brought in different bandages and talked about the various wound care options they could use. The typical dressing made my skin break out in a bubbly rash. That meant she had to come up with a plan B, which seemed to excite her even more. She made it seem as though the incision draining was the best thing that could've happened to her day. I had never met anyone more enthusiastic about wound care.

The doctors swarmed me the next day to give me the "fun" news from a CT scan that my sternum and surrounding area were infected and that I was soon to be off for another surgery. They were concerned about how my lungs would handle being put under since the anaesthetic medications are hard on the body. But they were so much more worried about the newly discovered massive infection in my chest that it was worth the risk.

I was sent down for surgery around 5:00 P.M. that day. It was the first time I had been in the OR while conscious and it was not comfortable. First of all, the place was freezing, and while they layered on the heated blankets, I could not get warm. Secondly, all the staff kept talking over each while they reviewed what was about to happen. They got my weight wrong (they had my old weight listed, but I had lost a lot of weight since the transplant), so I was slightly concerned that they were going to overdose me on the anaesthetic. I tried to tell them that the number was wrong, but no one was listening to me.

It was also weird to me that while the nurse was halfway through reviewing the surgery, the main surgeon interrupted her to ask what time it was and if they had officially started the clock. It felt as though he was more concerned about needing an exact time for the surgery start than knowing what he was supposed to do. I'm sure it's one of those medical procedures that makes sense to the staff, but it was not comforting as the patient. One of the last phrases I heard before the sedatives knocked me out was, "Surgery is beginning, start the clocks." While I was trying to process why everything seemed like a race against time, I was out.

I awoke back in the Step-Down Unit with two new lines attached to me. After removing one centimetre of my sternum, the doctors set up what's called a vacuum-assisted closure (vac) machine and a new chest tube for the extra drainage. The vac machine is apparently the latest technology in wound care, using negative pressure wound therapy. Basically, it suctions out all the moisture in the area so that the wound stays as dry as possible, letting the bottom tissue heal first. The focus of my care quickly switched from my new lungs—they were doing well—to the wound and the vac machine. The infection swabs that the doctor did eventually showed that it wasn't a bacterial infection, which was good news. They thought it may have been fungal, so they started me on an anti-fungal to ensure that it wouldn't return. Once the infected skin and bone had been removed, the procedure left me with exposed bone and quite a hole in my chest. I was annoyed that I had such a giant wound and was attached to yet another line, but I also found the entire thing fascinating.

With a traditional dressing, the area would have been packed with gauze to soak up the drainage and would need to be changed multiple times a day to keep the site as dry as possible. The multiple changes with traditional dressing would mean a higher risk of another infection as well as a higher risk of pieces of gauze getting stuck under the skin. The idea of gauze getting stuck in my body is something that still makes my skin crawl. The nurses were usually careful when it came to changing the gauze they had to use around my incision, but one day before the wound surgery, some gauze did get stuck under my skin. A doctor had looked at the transplant incision, removed the bandage, and then repacked the area with a somewhat ridiculous amount of gauze and tape. When the wound care nurse came to inspect the site a few hours later, she had a fit as the doctor had used a type of gauze that tended to flake off into little pieces. And flake off it had. As she ripped off the copious amounts of tape from my sensitive skin and pulled a thread from under my skin in an area that wasn't even infected, we both cursed that doctor and it instilled in me a fear of loose threads getting lost in my body. After that, any time a doctor or nurse would inspect the wound post-infection surgery and then pack in gauze as a temporary fix, I would ask whoever removed it next if they got all the pieces, even if it was on for only a few minutes. I was so paranoid.

The dressing for the VAC machine involved no gauze and seemed straightforward to me, even though all the nurses seemed terrified to change it. The machine was on continuously, which meant there was always a slight amount of pressure with tiny vibrations going through me. I would notice it more at night, while lying down, or when I was tired. It felt as though I was having continuous mini chest percussions. As the weeks wore on, I didn't notice it as much but could never completely ignore it. The dressing itself was changed every other day. The wound care nurse kept telling me how painful the dressing change would be and encouraged me to take pain medication before dressing changes. I had a pain pump for the first twenty-four hours after the surgery, which helped even though it made me feel groggy and nauseous. I had been told I would have a pain pump after the transplant surgery, but I think I was in a coma for so long—four days—that I didn't need it once I woke up.

Honestly, the worst part about the VAC machine was the tape being ripped off. Even then, unless the previous nurse had been overzealous with the tape, it wasn't intolerable, mostly because, at the time, I had no feeling around my incision. All the nerves had been cut and had not yet regrown. It was painful only when they would clean and poke near the exposed bone while asking, "Does this hurt?" It was more an odd, anxiety-inducing sensation to have people poke around at exposed areas without feeling it or being able to see what was happening.

I was hoping to sleep most of the day following the latest surgery (which also happened to be my birthday) in an attempt to recover, but in the morning before the nurses switched shifts, my night nurse informed me that, as I hadn't peed since the surgery, they were putting a catheter back in. I was not pleased and since I had no urge to go, suggested that maybe I just didn't have to. She gave me a look and pointed out that since I was being pumped full of liquids, of course my bladder was full.

I proposed instead that maybe I had just been dehydrated and I was absorbing all the fluids. To her credit, she didn't call me delusional and to appease me, she brought in an ultrasound machine to check how much liquid was in my bladder. The ultrasound confirmed her stance; a catheter needed to go back in. I tried everything to urinate on my own first, but I simply couldn't. Apparently, this is a common side effect of the anaesthetic medication, which causes the bladder to relax so much there is no response to stimulant signals.

Catheters were one of the medical procedures that made my skin crawl. I have no idea why, but even before the transplant, whenever I thought about the surgery, I would get squeamish about the fact that I would need a catheter. It was the last thing I wanted to deal with. And now I was about to need a second one. This time it was put in while I was awake. In the end, it was not a comfortable experience but wasn't as bad as I had built it up to be in my mind. As the nurse said, my bladder

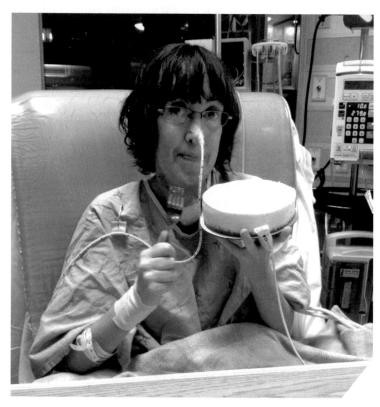

Allison celebrated her twenty-eighth birthday on December 30, 2014, in the Step-Down Unit at the Toronto General Hospital, after surgery for an infection in her sternum. Eating was a challenge post-transplant and it was a relief to be able to enjoy solid food once again. Meal replacement drinks were pumped through the nasal tube to help provide enough calories during her stay. (Isaiah Jacques)

was very, very full and it needed to be emptied. Happy twenty-eighth birthday to me.

The other big news of the day was that I was being moved down to the seventh floor—general transplant! My lungs and vital signs were stable, so I no longer needed such intensive nursing care. I was perplexed because I had just gotten out of surgery the previous day and didn't expect to be "kicked out" so quickly. Really, I just wanted a day to sleep. The nurses took down all the Christmas and birthday cards I had taped to the wall (I had so many cards mailed to me during my hospitalization—the amount of emotional and financial support I received from my community during the transplant was astonishing), threw all my belongings into hospital bags, handed me my birthday balloons, and whisked me off to the seventh floor.

16

ONE LITTLE BLOOD VESSEL

Being on the seventh floor, also known as general transplant, was quite a change from the Step-Down Unit. For starters, I had an excessively loud roommate, which was something new. One of the few advantages of having CF arises from hospital policies that give patients with CF private rooms to avoid the spread of germs. Moreover, my section of the shared room was tiny. There was a bed, chair, and small table all crammed together with barely enough room for a visitor. It was impossible to have two visitors at a time in the room. If Isaiah and another person visited, we would usually end up going to the family room. Finally, the nursing ratio was technically four to one, but once again someone always seemed to be on break, so it was realistically an eight-to-one situation. That meant far less hands-on care, which also meant I was expected to do most things for myself now.

It was a draining shock at first but pushed me physically, which was good in the long run. I had to wander down the hall to get my own ice chips, and I had to haul myself to the tiny bathroom. I had no one standing over me to get meals ready when the food arrived or to fetch my snacks from the communal fridge. It was all up to me. And it was all quite taxing. Although honestly, my visitors would often get what I needed, even though I protested, "I need to do it myself!" as I made no effort to move. I spent the first few days stunned by how tiring it was to do anything, like go to the washroom, but overall my endurance slowly increased.

Despite the setback of the infection of the transplant incision, I was eating much better since the removal of the trach, and the nurses on the seventh floor were determined that I would be taking my own pills. They didn't listen to my complaints and gave me loads of applesauce in which to put my pills. It was tedious taking one pill at a time because I was used to being able to swallow a handful at once. Slowly, I improved. My appetite increased daily, and while I was still getting nightly feeds through my nasal tube, I was eating more and more by myself. When I started getting more and more demanding about the food my visitors brought me, I took it as a sign that my health was improving.

Consistent with the other changes on the seventh floor, I was now expected to be up and walking on my own instead of waiting for a physiotherapist. I was moved from the standing walker to a regular walker, which was much easier to use. The physiotherapists checked on me every once in a while, but that was more to see how my tailbone was healing than to take me for a walk.

Isaiah or Mom (she returned right after New Year's) would walk little loops with me, either pushing the IV pole (when I was on antibiotics) or the walker with the VAC machine.

In the first week on the seventh floor, as the medical team had promised, I officially made the transition to no oxygen, which was surreal. In fact, the first time I went for a walk without oxygen was an accident. Isaiah and I decided to go around the nurses' station and halfway across the ward, I realized we had forgotten to bring my oxygen. That's when I realized I was finally comfortable without the extra support. I still kept checking my stats every so often over the next few days because I couldn't believe my lungs were holding steady with a 95% oxygen saturation on room air.

The VAC machine continued doing its healing thing, and there was some talk of discharging me. I was only cautiously optimistic. I had been hospitalized enough to know that there is no point believing anyone who mentions discharge until a nurse is pulling out the IV and giving you the discharge papers while a cleaner stands by anxiously waiting for you to leave so they can rid the room of your germs.

In the meantime, my VAC dressing was scheduled to be changed every Monday, Wednesday, and Friday. The first week I moved to the floor, somehow the dressing change got pushed back from the Friday to the Saturday. My Friday nurse kept saying that she couldn't do it because the orders hadn't come in yet from the wound care nurse, even though it had been changed by people on that floor on Wednesday. Her resistance was puzzling, and it occurred to me that she simply didn't want to deal with it. Either way, the dressing was changed on Saturday and was less painful than the previous time. I had no concerns while it was happening and I watched saline and blood pieces be suctioned through the tubing into the machine.

All was well until about midnight, when I noticed that blood was leaking from the site. I rang the night nurse who wasn't terribly concerned. She simply reinforced the tape with more tape. She figured the day nurse had gone overboard with the rinsing during the dressing change: it had irritated my skin enough for some minor bleeding, and this was the extra coming out. I thought it seemed like a delayed reaction, but since it was normal for the machine to sometimes pump out some blood, I assumed she knew what she was talking about and went back to sleep.

I woke up twenty minutes later to see that the leaking had soaked through both the new tape and my gown. I rang the nurse who spent the following hour trying to contain the leak by adding progressively different and more types of tapes and gauzes to the site. She would say it was sealed until I would ring five minutes later having bled through yet another johnny shirt and the protective bed pads. I went through a slew of shirts and sheets while she tried to contain the bleeding. She did everything possible to not change the bandage as it was considered a two-person job and she didn't have anyone to help out. Eventually, she declared victory and I drifted back to sleep.

I awoke to the sound of a loud beeping a few hours later and glanced down at my chest, only to realize I had been shot or, you know, the VAC dressing had started leaking through yet another gown. This time it made a perfect bloody circle on my chest. I started getting concerned at that point. The nurse, who by then had already arrived on the scene due to the high-pitched screeching coming from the machine, was not pleased at this new development.

My nurse brought in a back-up nurse and they both thought it was hilarious that it looked like I had a gunshot wound on my chest. They kept remarking how funny it would be to put it on Instagram and to say that I had been shot at the hospital. I was thinking it would be more fun if I could get cleaned up and go back to sleep. At last, they decided it was time to change the entire dressing. They shut off the screeching machine and went to work. However, once they started removing the layers of tape, they realized the bleeding was beyond their control. They called in extra reinforcement. Reinforcement, that is, the head nurse, took off the upper taping and decided to call in the resident. The resident, who glanced at the site and the amount of blood I had lost both on the bed and in the VAC machine, decided to call the surgeon. And the blood bank.

At this point, I was getting nervous because I didn't like the idea that no one would deal with the bleeding from the giant wound on my chest until the surgeon arrived. While we waited for him to get out of bed and arrive at the hospital, the nurses ran around like mad, emptying my tiny room of any unnecessary furniture (my one chair), taking loads of blood work to see what else was happening with me, continuously cleaning up the blood that seemed to be everywhere at this point, then taking more blood work when they thought of something else that should be tested.

By now, the tape was gone, but it appeared that no one wanted to be the one to remove the foam to see what was really happening with the wound until the surgeon arrived. That left my mind to wonder about worst case scenarios. In an attempt to comfort me, the nurse said that it could all be taken care of back in the OR and that sometimes people need to go back to have the infected skin removed a second time. My freaking out escalated to another level. I didn't want to go back to the OR. I couldn't handle that.

To my own amazement, I managed to doze off. When I opened my eyes again the surgeon was in the room and ready to make his assessment. (He had been called in from his house, and it was apparent that he was not thrilled to be there.) He had no qualms about removing the dressing and poking around the wound area. Thankfully the wound wasn't filled with blood as feared, but there was still some bleeding. He was able to determine that I was bleeding from a small site. The chaos resumed with people rushing in and out of my room getting various equipment so the surgeon could try to stop the bleeding. It was all a bit much. Part of the reason the chaos seemed so dramatic was the size of the room. It felt cramped when there was more than one person there at a time, so to have a surgeon, resident, head nurse, night nurse, and float nurse all in the room and all making suggestions, I started to feel overwhelmed and panicked. The head nurse looked at my file and said, "It says you have some history of anxiety attacks. This is an anxious moment, so you're getting medication." And so I was drugged up. I didn't even have to ask.

The surgeon continued to poke around the wound to find the cause of all the blood. It was uncomfortable, so the head nurse declared that I needed more pain medication. (No complaints from me.) I was swiftly connected to another IV and had some of the hallucinogenic pain medication pushed through my system. I was suddenly quite relaxed.

The source of the bleed was just a blood vessel, and it stopped once some pressure was applied. Turns out the nurse was partly right about my skin becoming irritated during the dressing change, causing the bleeding. Due to the nature of the VAC machine, the bleeding couldn't clot normally as the suction was continuously applied. Once the VAC machine was off and the suction was no longer there, the blood vessel could clot. I did not have to go back to the OR for a second wash, and there was no need for any other intervention. The surgeon put regular gauze on the site and decided it would all be reassessed in the morning. Problem solved.

Everyone cleared out, a unit of blood arrived from the blood bank to replenish all that I had lost, and I started slipping into a stoned sleep. I was prepared to have a pleasant medication-induced rest, except that I had been given the hallucination medication. Instead of a relaxing sleep, I kept waking up, thinking people were in my room to further treat my wound. I would open my eyes and the people would disappear, but as soon as I closed my eyes, they would return. My brain couldn't make the connection that the people couldn't be real if I only saw them when my eyes were closed. At one point I pressed the call bell for no reason I can explain other than I wanted to tell someone about the people in my room. A nurse came in, and I told him I was seeing people when I closed my eyes.

He asked, "Do you see them now?"

I responded indignantly, "Of course not, my eyes are open. They're only there when I close my eyes."

He slowly backed out of the room.

I later woke up in a panic that I couldn't breathe and started madly pressing the call button while hyperventilating. It took me a few minutes to realize that if I could hyperventilate, I was probably breathing. By the time the nurse showed up again, I apologized and told him that I thought I was stoned and making poor decisions. He agreed.

I eventually passed out in a calm sleep for a few hours. I woke up when the nurse came in to change my feeds and noticed that there was once again blood everywhere. The blood was much darker and less scary looking to me, but that was probably because I was still stoned. However, the nurse panicked—until she realized that the source of the mess wasn't my wound but my arm. Whoever was supposed to attach the blood to my IV hadn't connected it fully; instead of going into me, it went all over the bed. The head nurse was called again because she was the one who had to approve another unit of blood being sent up. She was furious that the blood had spilled and that she needed to call the blood bank again. I thought that heads were about to roll as she yelled at the other nurses to find out who was responsible.

Eventually the drugs wore off, I actually got the unit of blood to replenish my body, and the VAC machine was reattached the next afternoon with no problems. It had been a chaotic night of panic, all due to one irritated little blood vessel.

17

SOMEONE ELSE'S
LUNGS INSIDE OF ME

Once the bleeding drama was allayed, I had a few quiet days with the VAC machine pumping away uneventfully. I was informed that it was finally okay to have a shower. I was instructed not to linger, but because the VAC machine formed a tight seal around my wound, it would be kept dry so showering was permissible. While it took a lot of effort and was exhausting, a shower was also marvellous. I thought I might swoon from the joy of feeling truly clean for the first time in over a month. Although I still had so little strength that I only had energy to shower every few days, every time was as good as the first.

I was feeling mostly recovered and ready to start thinking about leaving the hospital. The only thing keeping me in the hospital was the giant wound on my chest. I was referred to the plastic surgeons to see if they could do anything to encourage the wound to heal faster. The doctors also didn't want to discharge me without the wound being stable for a few days: the "night of the blood" made them jumpy.

My new lungs were stable, and apart from some minor fluid issues and the fact that I couldn't cough effectively, it was smooth sailing. I admit that I didn't spend much time thinking about it. I was still in shock from everything that had happened around the transplant and I was blocking out the emotional side of the procedure. My focus was trained on getting through each day at the hospital, trying to get healthier and stronger. Figuring out what I needed to do to leave the hospital took all of my energy, so I didn't have any to spare to be emotional about all the new changes.

In the aftermath of my double-lung transplant, there always seemed to be something else of higher importance than my lungs; they were not my primary focus. Sounds strange, I know. It was odd that after such a long time of thinking only about my lungs, they had become a secondary concern. This was not only because of all the complications I was dealing with, but also because, for the first time in ages, I no longer *had* to think about them. I was on room air and able to breathe comfortably. My oxygen saturation held steady at 95–97%, which blew my mind. I didn't even notice how little I was coughing—not that I had the muscles to cough—until Mom mentioned how extraordinary it was that I could walk around the little hospital block without hacking. It was effortless to breathe for the first time in years. It was, and still is, hard to wrap my mind around the difference between before and after the transplant. I can breathe without stress. I no longer have to think about it every time I climb a flight of stairs or run across the road. The transplant literally saved my life—all because a family decided that their loved one would be an organ donor.

Organ donation differs emotionally from receiving blood or platelets, both of which I've received plenty of. With a blood transfusion, you know the person that donated the blood is still walking around somewhere. They spent an hour or two being uncomfortable and then carried on with their life. It's hard to think about the organ donor who died. It's easy to feel grateful toward the donor but difficult to contemplate who they were as a person. As part of the support group sessions, every few months they discussed any guilt or anxiety people felt about having the body parts of another person. I don't know if many people had trouble with this because I wasn't able to go to the support sessions, but it seemed to be talked about enough that it must've been an issue for some recipients.

Personally, I found the weirdest part about the whole experience was the "needing someone to die in order for me to live" part. I found it especially uncomfortable when people said they were praying for me to get lungs because it was difficult not to see that as praying for someone else's death. I know that was not the intent of these people, but it seemed like while they were praying for me to get lungs, another family was hoping that their loved one would wake up from a coma. This is something that I still have to detach myself from emotionally, although I contemplate it from time to time. It's complicated to know that the reason I'm alive is that someone else died. I found the notion especially uncomfortable around Christmas, when people at physiotherapy would make well-meaning comments about Santa delivering lungs, or would wish for a Christmas miracle. I couldn't stop thinking about how those wishes meant that some other family would have a loved one die around the holidays.

Pragmatically, I know that when I was wishing for a transplant, that didn't mean I was actively wishing for another person to die. I know that I was benefitting from someone else's death and I wasn't the cause of their death, but it still made me feel weird while hoping for the transplant. As the waiting year wore on, different months would make me think of who might be dying that month. I couldn't help wondering if I would get the transplant around June due to teenagers out partying after prom or graduation, or in November with the unexpected icy roads, or in the spring with the increased rate of suicides. I would think about it and then immediately feel bad but still hopeful that maybe I would get my lungs that month. Complicated.

Due to the Trillium Gift of Life Network Act in Ontario, the entire process is anonymous, although there are stories of people finding each other. (It's not anonymous in the United States, so people there tend to know their donor.) It's a lot easier to track people down these days thanks to the internet. My transplant happened around the time that former Toronto Maple Leafs coach Pat Quinn died, so my family had a crazy theory that I ended up with Pat Quinn's lungs and that meant, illogically, that I would become a hockey coach. (My family was pretty tired the first week of my surgery.)

But I do wonder who my donor was and how old they were when they died. And how they died. Would they be okay with the fact that I got their lungs? Was there anywhere they wanted to visit? Was their family happy they were an organ donor? I have so many questions that I don't think will ever be answered.

The Trillium Gift of Life Network provides an optional service for the donor family and recipient, allowing letters to be exchanged between the individuals. However, due to the Act requiring everything to remain anonymous, the letters can't include my name or any identifying features about me, nor can I receive any identifiers if the family wishes to contact me. The

Network strongly encourages recipients to write even a simple note of thanks to the family some time during the first year because it can help the family in their grief.

I put off writing the letter for as long as possible because every time I sat down to write something, I ended up crying instead. Eventually, with my six-month post-transplant anniversary approaching, I knew I had put it off long enough. I was thinking that by then I would be able to just jot down something, but it was still emotional. Every time I started the letter, I decided the dishes needed doing at that moment. A thank you note seemed so inadequate. How do you find the right words to express gratitude for being alive?

I did eventually write something because I figured the family would appreciate hearing that their decision not only saved my life but brought me a quality of life that I had hardly been able to imagine pre-transplant. I don't know if I'll ever receive anything back from the donor family but that's okay. It will always be one my life's great mysteries. Who knows, maybe it's best left up to my imagination, because that way I can picture the donor being whoever I want. But, no, I don't believe it was Pat Quinn.

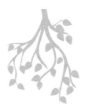

18

TRYING TO BREAK OUT
OF THE HOSPITAL

On January 7, 2015, I had the last line removed from my face when my nasal tube was taken out. I still had the VAC machine, drainage tubing, and PICC line, but it was another line down in the count toward freedom of all lines. When the nasal tube was in, every once in a while I would feel it in the back of my throat even though the doctors kept telling me I shouldn't and that it was mostly psychological. When I felt it in my throat, my reflexes would kick in and try to swallow it, and when I couldn't, I would feel as though I was choking. I found the nasal tube made it harder to eat because food would sometimes get stuck on the line. It was also a nuisance having something dangling in front of my mouth. All to say it was getting increasingly uncomfortable, and I was elated to have it gone. Now I was officially responsible for my own caloric and pill intake.

The strangest unexpected part was that after the nasal tubing came out, my first thought was, *I can't breathe*, and I started to panic. My brain eventually kicked in and realized that my thoughts made no sense as it was a feeding tube, not oxygen tubing. Somewhere along the line, the pressure from something in my nose had become so associated with oxygen that even a feeding tube made my brain think it was receiving oxygen. The mind is a funny thing. Once I convinced my lungs that they did not, in fact, need help from a feeding tube in order to get air, it felt freeing to have the tube out. My skin was able to start healing after a month of tape and lines. Hospitals are not good for skincare.

The absence of any lines down my throat eased pill swallowing. With the help of applesauce, I was able to swallow the small pills whole while the rest were still broken up. At one point, I reflexively put four digestive enzymes in my mouth at once and was prepared to swallow until I realized what I was doing and spit them all out. My old habits were trying to kill me. Pill swallowing gradually improved until I was able to swallow them without applesauce and then slowly worked up to two at a time. It was necessary to combine the pills as much as possible. With about fifteen pills each morning, it meant that I would be full from applesauce before I had even started eating breakfast. I was on a soft food diet for a long time, but that was okay as the only foods to avoid were anything stringy, raw, or seedy. The cheesecake that my family kept bringing in was definitely allowed.

The next big step was to return to the treadmill room to start with regular outpatient physiotherapy again. I was ready to get some muscles back and walking around the ward wasn't cutting it for me anymore. This is not something that usually happens with lung post-transplant patients. Most people are discharged by the time they can walk twice around the ward. In fact, that is one of the criteria for being discharged post-transplant. People start at physiotherapy again as outpatients. However, as it was my wound complications that were keeping me in the hospital and not my lungs or endurance, the doctors figured I might as well start exercising in earnest since everything else was going well.

It was almost scary how excited I was to get my green card (you may recall that yellow is pre-transplant and green is post-transplant). Even with everything I had been through, somehow holding the green card made the fact that I survived the transplant more real. I couldn't do much with my arms because the physiotherapists were concerned about stretching messing up my incision and/or VAC dressing, but I could manage all the leg work. And boy, was that enough. I walked slowly on the treadmill for twenty minutes and did some leg weights with a whopping three pounds. My vital signs stayed steady, and I may have coughed three times. I was tired but happy to be back. The hardest part was doing modified squats. Instead of regular squats, the physiotherapist had me "simply" stand up from a chair ten times. I thought my legs were going to give out, and that was with using my arms to help push myself off the chair. It was frustrating to have lost so much muscle mass, but I was determined that I would return to squats soon.

Discharge planning began in earnest on January 9, 2015. I had to have a medication training session with a pharmacist, as well as watch several informational videos and listen to a spiel from the discharge coordinator before I could go home. My PICC line was removed because it wasn't being used and kept getting blocked, which was creating a high risk of getting another blood clot. The drainage line for my wound was also removed. I only had the VAC machine left and knew that would be around for a while. The good news was that the team decided I could go home with it.

The medication training was straightforward. I, along with the four older men in my session, received brown bags of our medication with a booklet. The pharmacist reviewed every medication and its side effects, scaring us with all the horrible side effects the medications can cause. She also went over the signs of infection and rejection. And just like that, I was responsible for self-medicating while in hospital (under the strict supervision of a nurse, of course). I watched the informational videos with Mom and Isaiah. The videos simply reviewed what to look for with infection and rejection. Be alert for rashes! Go to an emergency department if you get a fever! Don't have open wounds! There were also reminders to eat properly, exercise regularly, and not be around sick people or strong chemicals.

The meeting with the discharge coordinator involved still more instructions on ways to spot infection and rejection. The entire discharge process seemed to be one giant lecture about washing hands, limiting hugs and handshakes, staying away from crowds, and treating everyone as though they had the plague. I have never been as cautious as I should have been when it comes to infection control, but I am much more paranoid since having the transplant, which, while not turning me into a hypochondriac, has made me much more aware any time anyone around me sniffles or coughs.

The days in the hospital wore on as I was supervised taking medication, continued attending physiotherapy, and ate better and better every day. I was starting to get restless, which I took as a sign that it was time for me to leave. At first I was drugged enough that I was content with little entertainment and I had my family around for most of the day. Everyone was there for the first week post-transplant, but eventually they had to return to their jobs. Amy and Dad stayed for another few weeks and Mom stayed for as long as she could. Isaiah's family also visited, as well as a few friends and cousins. The company really helped pass the time.

I had my family bring in some easy knitting to do and we played endless games of Wizard, Five Crowns, and other card games. I also had them bring in some of my art supplies and we made thank-you cards for everyone we knew. The only thing I usually did that I wasn't able to do in the hospital was read. I'm not sure if it was the new medication or the new environment, but I was not able to concentrate on a book, even if it had a light, silly plot. I've always been a reader; everyone in my family reads and usually has a book on the go, so it was a surprise that when I had downtime, I didn't turn to books. I think I was sleeping so much that it was hard to focus. I did, however, listen to a lot of podcasts. They were my book substitutes and told me stories without me having to focus on anything in particular.

December 28 had been the first day since the transplant (that I was conscious) that I didn't have a visitor by the afternoon. Isaiah was seeing his sisters off to the train station and my friend, who was in the city for a few days, had other people to visit. I am blessed to have so many friends and family who love me enough to sit by my side while I slept on and off, day after day, playing the same games, answering the same questions, and hanging out in a hospital every day. I never would've survived the trach-masking experience without Mom and Isaiah sitting beside me to play games and make countless cards with/for me. It would've been hell without them. Thanks everyone!

At the hospital, everything was looking ready for discharge by the end of the week when the plastic surgeons showed up to say surgery might be the best option for the wound to heal properly. I didn't want another surgery. I just wanted to go home. I was in going-home mode, and while I never fully got my hopes up, I was getting antsy about still being in the hospital. I didn't want to go back to the cold operating room or be afraid of dying from anaesthetic or have another IV or spend any more time in the hospital with its lack of privacy and single-ply toilet paper and a roommate who never stopped screaming. I wanted my own bed, dammit! But I didn't outright refuse because if another surgery meant a faster healing process for my wound, ultimately it would be worth it. The plastic surgeons made a good case for the surgery and scheduled me for a CT scan so they could evaluate where my muscles were and what they would have to work with if they tried to cover up the exposed bone area. The idea was that they would somehow find extra muscles in my chest, move them around, slap on a skin graft, put on the pressure VAC machine for a week or so, and voila: one healed wound.

I was stuck waiting for tests instead of packing to leave. My patience with the hospital food and my screaming roommate was wearing thin, in spite of the rationale for the delay. The VAC machine continued to suck up goo from the wound. Stupid wound.

When I went for my CT scan the next day, it turned out that the communication in the forms was crossed. I ended up having a regular CT scan despite the nurse telling me I was supposed to have the one with the dye injection. I informed the technicians that they were doing the wrong scan but they responded that they couldn't do anything other than what the form directed and refused to call the floor to make sure they were doing the right test. It was a giant waste of time.

As a result of the screw-up, the next day I had to go for the proper CT scan with dye, which meant that I needed an IV big enough for the dye to go through. Since my PICC line had been removed, they had to put in a new line. That was going to be difficult because by now, both of my arms were completely bruised and all my veins were tapped out. It was a struggle every morning for people to draw blood from me, and putting in an IV is much more difficult than drawing blood.

I knew I was about to become a pin-cushion and dreaded everything about it. Several nurses tried various spots on my arms with no luck. Each nurse is allowed to try twice and they are supposed to rotate through every nurse on the floor before calling in back-up from another floor (usually they call in an anaesthetist because they put in IVs all the time). They didn't go through every nurse on the floor, but it seemed like many tried. I was in pain after being poked so often and wondered whether the CT scan was worth it. Then a doctor walked into my room determined that she would be the one to put in the IV.

She put the tourniquet super-tight to cut off all circulation (it was necessary), and after one failed attempt, went for a small vein in the back of my hand. She got the needle in the vein which was excellent. What wasn't excellent was that she hadn't prepped the needle by attaching the closing cap with flush. Due to the nature of the IV, the line was open, allowing blood to gush all over her, me, and the bed. She seemed bewildered about what was happening and screamed for a nurse.

One of the nurses had prepped everything on the table at the end of my bed but the doctor couldn't reach it while also trying to stop the blood flowing from my hand. She half-screamed at Mom, who was watching from the other side of the room in horror, to try to curb the blood flow. Mom ran over and applied pressure as the doctor tried to figure out how to cap off the IV.

A nurse eventually came to fix the problem, but not before I bled all over the bed, floor, Mom, and the doctor. The doctor mumbled something about at least it was now in and left the room to wash up. She came back later and said that they use different IVs in the UK where she did her training so that's why she wasn't prepared. It was a bloody case of a doctor trying something that she probably hadn't done since medical school. To me, it was clear she had no idea how to use that particular equipment.

Once the IV was in, I was whisked off to CT once again for the dye scan. The scan went smoothly, but I didn't hear anything from the plastics team for days. Discharge planning was on hold and the transplant team wouldn't say boo without talking to plastics first. While waiting, Isaiah, Amy, and I played games, went for walks, and generally tried not to lose our minds.

By the following Wednesday, I was told that the plastics team had decided not to operate. The head plastic surgeon looked at my wound, poked around, and confirmed that it was healing nicely on its own with the VAC machine. He didn't think I had enough muscle for what they wanted to do or that I seemed strong enough for another surgery. He mentioned a skin graft to help it finish healing but was vague about it. That never happened either; in fact, I never heard from the plastics team again.

As the plastics team was the only thing keeping me in the hospital, I was itching to leave that day, but there were some complications with my paperwork concerning the portable VAC machine. While I waited for the paperwork to be sorted out, I met with my post-transplant coordinator who provided me with loads of paperwork and follow-up appointments. The next day I thought I was going home because homecare was arranged, medication was ordered from the pharmacy, and goodbyes had been said by all. However, my body revolted: I felt nauseous, started vomiting, and my heart rate spiked while walking to physiotherapy. The feeling continued for the rest of the day so no one felt comfortable discharging me. I was beyond frustrated but at the same time, it was hard to argue when I was curled around a barf basin in bed.

On Friday, January 23, 2015, it looked like discharge might be the real deal. The doctors were concerned about the possibility of me having an infection because one of my cultures showed something might be growing. They said I may need to return but that I could flee for the night while they waited for the results. I agreed. Anything to go home.

I was all set to go, had my discharge papers, was switched to the portable VAC machine, and Isaiah had carted my belongings off to the car, only to have my nurse come in right after saying, "Pack up!" to say, "Just one dose of IV antibiotics before you go!" Of course, that involved putting in a new IV which meant two nurses and five stabs before they could get one into my bruised veins. After that went on for many torturous hours, I was finally let go around 6:30 P.M. The resident who signed me off was the same one I had had at St. Mike's pre-transplant and who had been on the night I was admitted to the TGH after I got The Call. It was fitting that he was the one who officially discharged me.

A transport wheeled me to the entrance where Isaiah waited with the car to drive me home. I breathed in fresh air (well, Toronto air) for the first time in almost two months. Seventy-six days after being admitted to St. Michael's. Fifty-eight days since having a double-lung transplant, three surgeries, GI bleeds, blood clots, a sternum infection and removal, wound bleeds, and blood transfusions. I was finally going home.

PART IV

HOME TO FINISH HEALING

FEBRUARY TO JUNE 2015

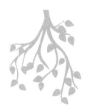

19

TRANSITION BACK HOME—TWICE

For all that I had been looking forward to returning home to our Toronto apartment, it was scary to be there. I wasn't sure if I was ready to be responsible for my own health. I had been in the hospital for so long with everyone else taking care of my appointments and medical decisions that the transition back to doing it all myself seemed staggering. I felt certain I was going to take a wrong medication or miss a follow-up appointment. I discovered the blood-thinner needles I had to inject myself with were terrifyingly large, and they weren't the only needles I had to use. I also had to give myself a daily insulin injection with smaller needles because my sugars were elevated from the steroid I had to take. Isaiah ended up giving me both injections every morning for a while because I was too intimidated to do it myself. I would ask him to inject me but then yell at him when it hurt, as though he should've, at some point, been trained to deliver needles painlessly. Since it hurt when the nurses gave them to me, I'm not exactly sure how I thought Isaiah would be able to deliver pain-free needles. This adjustment period was not a highlight of our relationship.

While it was overwhelming to be home after being in the hospital for so long, it was also heartening. I could finally do things on my own like make my own tea and have a brief soak for my dried-out legs. (I couldn't have a full bath because of the VAC dressing, but I could still shower and have half-baths.) On Saturday, January 24, when I was finally opening my Christmas stocking from my family and eating some delicious, homemade food, my phone rang. It was the hospital, informing me that I did indeed have an infection as they suspected and that I needed to go in immediately for some IV antibiotics. My time without visiting a hospital lasted a grand total of twenty-four hours.

I finished eating supper and then we drove to the emergency department. The nurses were not particularity pleased to see me and made it clear that I was wasting their emergency department time for some antibiotics. They struggled to get an IV in, but once they were successful everything else went smoothly. I sat in the waiting room while the medication ran through, playing the "why is everyone else here" guessing game. Once I had received the necessary medication, we returned home.

I went back to the emergency department on Sunday for more antibiotics. The doctor told me then that I would be contacted on Monday about what to do next. When Monday rolled around, I phoned the hospital after not hearing from anyone. I got a stern lecture from the doctor: "You were supposed to be here at 9:00 A.M. Where are you? Why aren't you here?" I apologized for the confusion and promised to go in first thing the next morning for an echocardiogram and blood work. It was luxurious to sleep in my own bed, and I was reluctant to give that up.

Around 3:00 A.M. Tuesday morning I woke with a sharp pain in my right arm. I tried to say something to Isaiah about how weird it felt but couldn't manage to get any words out. At that moment every muscle in my body seemed to seize at once with the most intense pain before I passed out. I woke up strapped to a stretcher and tried to ask what was happening before I felt the sharp pain again in my right arm. It moved to my entire body, causing me to again pass out.

It turns out I was having seizures.

I'm told that after the first seizure, Isaiah woke up (good thing he's a light sleeper) and immediately called 911. When the paramedics showed up, I had another seizure in bed. They wanted to take me to St. Mike's but Isaiah convinced them that the TGH was the best option for me as I had just been discharged from there. I had another seizure (the one I half-remember) when we first arrived at the emergency department and then another one once they transferred me to an actual bed. The doctors pumped me full of anti-seizure medication, putting my entire body in relax mode so I slept all of Tuesday. While I slept, they sent me for a CT scan and MRI to determine what was causing the seizures.

I was moved to the transplant Step-Down Unit where I had my own room, constant monitoring, and two-to-one nursing care. The results from the CT scan showed that I may have had a spot on my brain causing the seizures, so to be sure, they sent me back for a CT scan with dyes to get a better resolution. (I was still passed out for all of this.) The second CT scan was clear and showed no brain spotting. The spot on the first one must have been a glitch or a stain on the technician's computer. Hurray for no brain aneurism!

The doctors inferred the seizures were caused by one of my anti-rejection medications after my blood work report showed I had a "toxic" level of one in my system. My body was retaining the medication instead of breaking it down. Of course, they wouldn't say with 100% certainty that was the cause, but in my experience doctors rarely make such strong statements.

The anti-rejection medications I was on, and the different ones I am still on, have powerful side effects. Many of the medications I'm on are a reaction to the initial immunosuppressive medication. The steroid increases blood sugar levels, which means that I require insulin injections to counteract the effects. Others increase heart rate, so for a while, I needed a pill to counter that effect as well. It's a nasty cycle but one that I can't break because the initial reason for needing the anti-rejection medication will never change. It's a lifelong commitment, so I just have to deal with all the side effects, hopefully minus more seizures.

Once I woke up, my brain was foggy. I was grateful that Isaiah was around to explain why I was waking up in a hospital bed with only a johnny shirt on (seriously, where did my pyjamas go?), feeling like I had been run over by a truck. I was frustrated to be back in the hospital. It was a giant step backward in my recovery process. I barely had energy to stand up and kept getting head rushes whenever I tried, so I was clearly in no shape to go home. My jaw hurt because I must've clenched it during the seizures and my entire body was wiped. Having seizures is exhausting.

It took a few days for me to stop feeling dizzy if I moved my head too quickly or stood up too fast. No one could explain why I was so dizzy and they didn't know if it was from the new anti-seizure medication or a residual effect from the seizures. I was started on a new anti-rejection medication that didn't give me seizures, a pleasant change. I asked the doctor nicely if I could leave on the Friday since I hadn't had any more seizures and my medications seemed to be sorted out. My question was met with a snort and a resounding, "Not a chance in hell," so I grudgingly spent the weekend in the hospital. The transplant team wanted to monitor me for a few more days on the new medication before sending me off on my own. They also wanted me to see the neurologist (which didn't actually happen as an in-patient).

I was still on the antibiotics for the infection I had before I was discharged initially, and since my arms were black and blue from all the IVs and blood work, the team thought a PICC line was in order. A radiologist tried to put in the line in my room, but for some reason he couldn't thread the wire past my shoulder. Since the room didn't have an x-ray machine and he only had the ultrasound machine to work with, he gave up and put in a request for it to be done in a procedure room. We were both disappointed because it meant a weekend full of IVs and blood work pokes that were getting increasingly harder for the technicians to do successfully.

I was moved down to the seventh floor, which meant I was no longer attached to the ECG machine; however, it also meant I had less nursing care and a new roommate. The person was much quieter than my previous roommate (I doubt anyone could be louder). Over the weekend, I was moved to a private room—a pleasant surprise. Someone in administration thought that I needed a private room because of my infection. The nurses were all confused about the move, but I wasn't about to argue.

Things remained status quo for the week. I continued getting sick of hospital food. I had praised it at the start of my post-transplant experience but by the time I was on my sixth week of hospital food, I was ready for a change. Mashed potatoes and stringy roast beef no longer had the same appeal as when I was first allowed to start eating. And there seemed to be a two-week rotation of the menu. As a result, I ate a lot of onion rings from the fast-food places in the hospital food court. For some reason I never got as tired of those; deep-fried food somehow manages to remain delicious for days on end.

Every day of that week, the nurse would say, "Today is the day to leave!" but then something else would come up to keep me there. My anti-rejection levels were not increasing as quickly as the team wanted and the doctors were understandably concerned about hiking up the medication and sending me on my way. It was a balancing act between getting the levels to the appropriate amounts and making sure my body didn't go into shock. The team finally decided that they could monitor everything as an outpatient as long as I went in for blood work three times a week to have my levels checked.

On Friday, February 6, 2015, I was discharged for a second time from the TGH. After reviewing my blood work and making me promise to return on the following Monday morning, the doctors decided there wasn't anything else they could do for me in hospital. I was given my new medications with information about all the possible scary side effects and was finally set free.

The other news upon discharge was that the wound care nurse thought that I would only need the VAC machine and dressing for another week. Hurray! While the home machine was much more portable than the one I had in hospital, I was beyond ready to not be connected to anything. It was cumbersome to carry with me whenever I moved around the apartment. However, that didn't mean my wound was finished healing. The incision was still fairly large; it was just becoming too shallow for the foam to fit in properly. There was a risk that the foam could start irritating the healthy skin around the wound, which would set back the healing process. After a week, I hoped to be able to switch to a conventional dressing that was supposed to be much more convenient. I appreciated that the VAC machine had super healing speed, but it was uncomfortable. Isaiah and I celebrated my return home by watching TV and generally doing as little as possible. We hoped this time I could last longer than three days before being readmitted.

And I did!

I returned to the hospital for blood work and then to physiotherapy the following week. The seizures set me back physically though. Any muscle I had been rebuilding after my transplant quickly receded. It was unbelievably frustrating, but there was nothing I could do besides persevere to rebuild my strength. I had thought I would be further along in my recovery process by that point and was disheartened that I had suffered such a big setback. The infection I could deal with; it was the physical weakness after the seizures that was such a shock to my system. I became tired doing the simplest tasks; however, while it was discouraging, I was determined to get stronger. After all I had been through, I was not about to give up because of a few seizures.

After the seizures, being home was once again difficult. I kept trying to do more and more for myself but I was struggling just to find the energy to get dressed every morning, let alone help with the laundry. I felt that since I had my new lungs, I should immediately be able to start helping out with the housework again. However, another part of me just wanted to sit on the couch and let Isaiah continue to do everything. He grew tired of that rather quickly, and since I was technically healthy, he refused to wait on me hand and foot anymore. Pre-transplant, he had done all the housework while I contributed by cleaning the bathroom every once in a while. Post-transplant, he was ready for me to start helping out again. Not that he was harassing me to clean the apartment, he just felt I should be getting up from the couch to make my own cups of tea. Fair enough.

There is a fine line between being a supporter and being an enabler. Isaiah did remarkably well at pushing me to do as much as possible while recognizing that sometimes I simply didn't have the energy to get off the couch. It makes for a weird relationship when one person becomes the caregiver. It's hard for both people to switch from an egalitarian relationship to a much more dependent type of relationship. It was much easier to make the switch back to the egalitarian relationship, although I've heard that can also be challenging. After being a caregiver for so long, some people can feel lost when they no longer have a person to look after. I'm sure most couples experience changes in their relationship when someone gets the flu or food poisoning and one person ends up doing more around the house while the other sits on the couch eating soup. It was like that for us, only for months with no real end in sight.

My new routine at home became: three times a week, I would get up early and Isaiah would drive me to the hospital (I wasn't allowed to drive) to be stabbed for my precious blood. I would scarf down some food, take my medication, and suffer through physiotherapy. We would drive home, and I'd collapse on the couch for the rest of the afternoon. The first week back at physiotherapy after the seizures was tough. The tiny amount of stamina and muscle I had built up post-surgery seemed to have disappeared between the seizures and the two weeks I spent in the hospital. How is it that the body loses muscle mass so quickly but takes such a long time to build it?

I was exhausted all the time. I couldn't even complete the full fifteen minutes on the bike at physiotherapy and walked slowly on the treadmill. I didn't know if it was my body adjusting to the new medication or if I just needed to build up more muscle. Either way, I felt a general exhaustion most of the time, which got worse when I tried to push myself. My ten "sit-to-stands"— literally standing up from a chair ten times—made me feel as though I was going to fall over. It shouldn't have been that hard. I felt I had left all my leg muscles in the hospital bed during the previous two months.

Pre-transplant, I had this romantic idea that when I was post-transplant, the physiotherapists would be telling me not to push myself so hard for fear of overdoing it. I had heard them say those exact words to other people post-transplant, but when I expressed fear of overdoing it to the physiotherapist, she said that wouldn't be a problem. I was told to push myself as much as possible. I was so delusional about how post-transplant recovery was going to be. While I had tried hard pre-transplant not to imagine the post-transplant world for fear of hyping it up too much, I couldn't help but see other people post-transplant at physiotherapy and was always encouraged by how much progress they made. As for me, however, it seemed like I was spending all my time sleeping and trying to walk up a single step. It was great that I could breathe easily, but I was frustrated by my inability to do anything else.

The fact that I was still relatively early in my recovery process seemed irrelevant to my emotions. I wanted to be better instantaneously and didn't want to struggle anymore. The general exhaustion I felt was so different from my pre-transplant exhaustion that I was scared it would never leave. It's not as though I had a lot of energy before the transplant, but it was familiar and I knew how far I could push through it. Post-transplant was a different type of exhaustion. I'm still not sure whether it was because suddenly my limiting factor was my legs instead of my lungs. Perhaps it was because I felt like I should be doing more overall, whereas before I was okay with not being as capable because I knew there wasn't room for physical improvement. Maybe it was simply that I had lost a lot of weight and muscle mass and was less physically capable than I was pre-transplant, despite the fact that I could now breathe comfortably. Whatever the reason, I was happy to be able to return to physiotherapy to work on my muscles. Eventually I was able to accept that my body was still healing and with that came a lot of sleeping.

A milestone for me in February was purchasing a micro spirometer, a small hand-held device that records one's FEV1. I use the machine every morning by blowing into it three times and recording the best result. The first week I used it, my numbers were all over the place; however, the idea was that once the number stabilized and I was at my "max number," I'd be able to know my "normal" and to detect any change. Three days of decline and I'm supposed to inform the transplant team. It felt good to be able to concretely measure progress for a change.

My first few numbers ranged from a FEV1 of 0.50 to 0.90. I felt as though I was doing it wrong because my number pre-transplant was 0.70 and it made no sense that I could be 0.50 while feeling good and not needing oxygen. I met with my coordinator who reassured me that I was using the device correctly, even if the numbers were low. I was convinced that the machine ran low or that something was wrong, until I had my first official lung function test, which confirmed that my micro spirometer was correct.

My first official clinic appointment, on February 18, 2015, consisted of blood work, an x-ray, and pulmonary function tests (PFTs). My x-ray looked great, my blood work was fine, and my PFTs were horrible. I had to do the complete workup of tests, which was exhausting. It seemed official: my new lungs were not working as well as expected. They were about as bad as I could've imagined with a FEV1 of 0.87, or around 30% of my expected lung capacity. I would have been excited about that number pre-transplant, but I was hoping for much higher with better lungs. I panicked, ranting about the numbers to everyone in clinic because I had heard stories of people having more than 70% lung capacity post-transplant; I thought I should be as successful as them. However, everyone in clinic seemed relaxed about the readings and assured me that the numbers would improve as my body healed. It was all about strengthening the lungs. As I got stronger, the numbers would go up as well. They weren't concerned, so I tried hard not to be as well (although I secretly panicked continuously).

The medical people were right: my numbers did improve, not as much as 70–90% as I had hoped, but seemed to settle at a 65% range. My coordinator told me many times that the numbers can increase for the first year or so and to not to feel as though I'm stuck at this point. But I've plateaued and have come to accept it. My lungs were far from a perfect match and had to be cut down to fit my body. Because of that, combined with my bleeding and pulmonary embolism, it's amazing they worked at all. Lung capacity is not as important as staying stable and avoiding infections as much as possible. My oxygen saturation levels were excellent, my heart rate was fine, and I didn't feel short of breath. Clearly, something was working.

The other big step in February was that I was finally detached from the VAC machine. Homecare and the doctors had decided that the wound had healed enough to move to traditional dressings. I was finally free from any lines for the first time in over a year! No oxygen lines, no IV lines, no drainage tubes, no VAC dressing lines, just me wandering around in the world. It was satisfying to be able to walk without worrying if I was going to trip over tubing. I had become so accustomed to the oxygen line that I barely noticed it by the end, but I was much more paranoid about the VAC tubing. The oxygen tubing would just fall off my face if/when I tripped on the cord, but the VAC line had the possibility of pulling the dressing off my chest. I did stumble on it a few times, giving the tape a good tug, but the VAC tape held tight.

Of course, my wound was still serious. I moved to a "traditional dressing," which meant a layer of antimicrobial gauze with a fancy bandage slapped on top. It was much more comfortable and my chest no longer made weird hissing noises while I was trying to sleep. The downside was that I couldn't shower with the traditional dressing so I had to return to shallow baths and washing my hair in the sink. If I knew what time the nurse was arriving, I could have a quick shower immediately before, as it didn't matter if the bandage fell off at that point. The other downside to the traditional dressing was that I had daily nurse visits instead of every other day. It meant more waiting around for homecare, but daily changing of the dressing was much better for healing—and that was the goal.

20

THREE-MONTH
MILESTONE

The first week of March 2015, I had my three-month post-transplant assessments. They were more thorough than my regular clinic appointments, and the tests were spread out over several days because the three-month post-transplant mark is a significant milestone. It is usually when the transplant team discharges people from the outpatient program and gives the okay for them to return to their hometowns. People are most at risk for rejection, infections, and other complications during the first three months following transplant because the body is still healing. If people survive the first three months, there is a good chance they will make it to a year. After the three-month mark, a lot of the anti-rejection medications are lowered and most of the precautionary antibiotics are stopped.

At the three-month mark, I was able to stop the aerosol masks I had been on my entire life. Most people with CF stop them immediately post-transplant, but because of a bacteria that was in the transplanted lungs I received, the doctors wanted to try and eliminate it with an inhaled antibiotic before it could colonize further. Before the transplant, I had been on two aerosol masks plus chest percussions every morning and evening, so one mask twice a day was a treat. Stopping the masks completely was a luxury. I could wake up and get out of bed immediately. I no longer had to allocate a large chunk of time every morning before going anywhere. It was easy to drop it from my routine. I have been on aerosol masks since, as the bacteria flares up once in a while. Going back on daily aerosol masks is a pain but not something that I get stressed over. If having to do a mask a few times a year is the payment required for living, I'll take it.

During the assessments, the first test I had to get through on the Friday was the gastric-emptying study. It measures how fast the stomach can digest food. I have learned that some people have problems post-transplant with digestion because the nerves may have been impaired during surgery. The study checks to make sure that people are properly digesting their food. In preparation for the test, I had to fast for twelve hours and when I showed up, the technician plopped a breakfast of egg whites, toast laced with radioactive material (barium, I assume), and a tiny cup of water in front of me. I had ten minutes to eat the food and I was to drink as little of the water as possible. I struggled to get that food down. I barely had an appetite thanks to my antibiotics, and as it was, I wasn't much of a breakfast person at that point. (I sure am now!) I'm not sure anyone would enjoy dry, cold egg whites with toast at 8:00 A.M.

but add in a weird crunch thanks to the barium (remember, I hate weirdly textured food) and I almost threw up several times. I managed to get it down only because of the constant reminder playing through my brain that if I didn't eat it or if I threw it up, I would be back next week to do it all over again.

After consuming the terrible food, I stood in an x-raytype machine that was pressed around my abdomen and took a one-minute video of my stomach. The video x-ray was repeated on the hour, every hour, until I had less than 10% of the food left in my stomach. It took three hours for me, which meant being squished in the x-ray machine two more times. The long process was boring because they didn't want me doing anything in between that might affect the results, so I sat in a comfy chair and stress-knitted.

Some of the more standard medical appointments followed that initial test. I had my wound dressing changed at the outpatient clinic and did my six-minute walk test at physiotherapy. It was terrific to be able to do the walk test without dragging oxygen along, fearful of tripping over the tank or once again running over the physiotherapist's toes. (I did that only once.) However, I made it a total of 437 metres, which was less than my last pre-transplant walk of 548 metres. I did not take this news well. Even though I knew rationally that my body was not yet as physically strong as it was pre-transplant, I had hoped I would do better. I dislike seeing the evidence on paper that my body is physically weak. The positive part was that my oxygen levels stayed steady and my heart rate didn't shoot up. The not-so-positive part was that at about the three-minute mark, my legs were on fire, and at five minutes, I stopped feeling them. I'm not the best at pacing myself. I had actual physiotherapy after lunch followed by a CT scan. I was quite grumpy by the time I got home that day and napped for a few hours before I felt any better. I do not recommend scheduling a gastric-emptying test, wound-dressing change, six-minute walk test, physio, and CT scan all on the same day.

The following Monday, I had extra blood work, physiotherapy, and an x-ray. In the afternoon, I met with the transplant pharmacist—something I had never done outside of being an in-patient. When I was an in-patient and being discharged, the pharmacists showed up frequently to review medication and make any changes. The meeting as an outpatient proved to be almost the same thing. We reviewed my medication list and made some updates. The pharmacist warned me about any medication interactions. (No grapefruit for me.) She also heard all my complaints about the side effects I was having, like being shaky all the time, losing hair on my head, and having new hair growth elsewhere. She listened patiently and then told me there was nothing she could do. I would just have to live with the side effects of the medication.

I also had my PFTS on that visit, which took a long time because they seemed to want every test possible. It was exhausting. Each test is repeated a minimum of three times, more if I screw up or don't do well. As it's all computerized, the computer notes if an attempt is more than 10% off from the others and won't accept that one into the system. Consequently, it can take five or six times before there are three numbers in the 10% range. I felt as though I'd been through a full-body workout by the end.

The actual clinic appointment that day went quickly. I was running late thanks to my long lung function tests and most people had gone home already. I think the doctor wanted out of there as much as I did. There were no results from my gastric-emptying test but my CT scan looked better than the one from December (yay!). Apart from minor changes to a few of my medications, there wasn't anything else to review.

The next day was my last official "three-month assessment" procedure. It was the horrible twenty-four-hour pH study, designed to look at a person's acid reflux and heartburn post-transplant. I was told this study became necessary when people post-transplant, with no prior history of problems, would aspirate during the night and bronchoscopies would reveal food in their lungs. When they found enough food in enough people's lungs, they decided to test everyone for acid reflux as a proactive measure against aspiration pneumonia.

Understanding the reason for the testing did not make it any easier. A technician shoved a tube up my nose, threading it into my stomach. It was horrible. At least with the nasal feeding tubes, I was unconscious or semi-unconscious when it was put in. The insertion of the tube for the pH study may have been worse than the bronchoscopy in terms of ranking traumatic medical procedures. There was no sedation involved because it's supposedly a "super-easy" procedure. (Everyone lied to me!) Instead, a small amount of freezing gel was squirted up my nostril, but I'm not sure it helped.

It seemed as if it took hours for her to get the tube up my nose and into my stomach (Isaiah claims it was ten minutes at most), during which time I managed to throw up the small amount of water in my stomach, dry heave, and continuously gag while unsuccessfully holding back sobs and tears. Once it was finally in, I had to drink sips of "special apple juice" (as she called it) while she measured...something. I think it was a baseline pH level, but I'm not sure and frankly didn't care at that point. I was supposed to swallow the juice in one gulp and then relax my throat for several seconds. However, as my body was reflexively trying to get rid of the tube, I could not stop swallowing and gagging. I'm not positive she got any good results.

For the second part of the study, the first tube was pulled out and a second smaller one was inserted. The second tube went down much better, probably because it was smaller, but possibly because my nose and throat were too sore to notice. The second tube was then attached to a small machine that I carried around for the rest of the day and the following day. The machine had various settings that I would press any time I switched from "lying down" to "eating" or "sitting."

I was supposed to eat and drink normally to get an accurate recording but after that trauma, my appetite was shot for the day. It hurt to swallow or talk or to move my head too quickly. It was an unpleasant night, made worse by a call informing me of a scheduled bronchoscopy the following week. I was quite happy the next day to return the machine and have the tube removed, which was much less traumatic. I was promised that the study would never have to be repeated, so I'm holding them to that promise.

After my clinic testing, I had about a week to rest before I was due back in the hospital for my follow-up bronchoscopy and appointments. I had a friend from St. John's visit us in Toronto. It was St. Patrick's Day weekend, so we hit up the parade and ate some yummy food at different restaurants. Standing around for the parade was the first time I started to feel as though maybe my body would eventually feel better. It was also the first time that I took the streetcar/subway post-transplant which was exciting. These random "first times" were much more exciting than I ever expected they would be.

The confidence-booster continued during physiotherapy after the weekend. I felt physically strong for the first time in a long while. I was able to increase both my arm and leg weights, the treadmill speed, and during the much-hated sit-to-stand exercises, my thighs didn't give up on me at the end. It was a turning-point for my energy levels; after that weekend and physiotherapy on Monday, my energy improved.

My optimism lasted until that Wednesday, when I had another bronchoscopy. It was my second bronchoscopy as an outpatient and my first one was a terrible experience. During the first one, on February 19—the day after my first transplant clinic as an outpatient—my lungs were still quite weak, so the doctor was uncomfortable giving me lots of sedatives, on the grounds my body might not handle it well. She ignored my pleas to "take that chance anyway" and seemed to think I was joking. She told me they try not to knock people out completely but use just enough sedatives to put patients in a pleasant state so they are indifferent to the tube going down their throat. The nurse gave me some sedatives, which made me feel numb, but it turns out that the doctor was mistaken about people no longer caring about the tube.

I cared. I cared a lot. But I couldn't do anything because I was so out of it that my muscles weren't responding to my attempts to leap off the bed. It ranks among the worst experiences of my life.

No surprise, then, that I was having severe anxiety about a repeat experience when I discussed the bronchoscopy with the doctor during clinic the Monday before the procedure. The only thing that was keeping me relatively calm was that the doctor had said she could give me more sedatives because my lung function had increased. After being discharged from the hospital, my anxiety attacks had all but disappeared, except when it came to tubing being shoved into my lungs. The day of the procedure, I had been calm for most of the morning, and since my bronchoscopy was at 1:00 P.M., I had a lot of time to try not to panic. As we were driving up to the hospital, I got a call from the coordinator asking why I wasn't at my appointment. I responded that I was on my way and that it wasn't until 1:00 P.M. so I had plenty of time. She replied that, no, it was at 11:00 A.M., I was incredibly late, and the nurses were not pleased. Oops.

Isaiah dropped me off at the door and while he went to find parking, I rushed off to the second floor to get a lecture from the admitting nurse. I apologized, quickly changed, and moved to the gurney only to be lectured by the pre-operation nurse about leaving my list of medications in the car. I apologized again, saying that I was rushed and panicked when I left the car, and that my partner would be bringing it when he arrived in a few minutes. She scoffed and looked up the information on the computer even though Isaiah walked in a few minutes later with the medication list. Afterward, I got a lecture from another nurse about having had a small breakfast at 7:00 A.M. I replied that the doctor had said it was okay because my bronchoscopy wasn't until early afternoon and I would have had time to digest. She responded that "it was scheduled for 11:00 A.M.," to which I said, "Yes, but I didn't know that." So many lectures in so little time.

In the end, as the doctor waited impatiently outside of the room for the freezing aerosol to finish, the nurse told her that I had had breakfast and gave me a stare. The doctor said we had talked about it and that it was no problem. At least someone had my back. I think the stress may have helped me stay calmer because responding to angry nurses kept my mind off the actual bronchoscopy and focused on how terrible everyone was being. I was given more sedatives as promised, but I still didn't pass out as fully as I had wanted. I couldn't stop shaking, even though the nurse kept piling more and more blankets on me; I was shaking more from anxiety than the cold. Afterward, the doctor said it was a much harder procedure than the previous one. I found them both equally terrible.

One of my last major appointments in Toronto was to see the neurologist at the Toronto Western Hospital. It was the consultation that the doctors had booked after my seizures. Although they had told me that I may have to wait up to six months for the appointment, there was a cancellation, and I was in after about a month. The neurologist had me review what happened regarding the seizures. I tried to answer all of his questions regarding the events even though I was passed out the entire time. Afterward, I sat on the examination table and he tapped my arms and legs, testing my reflexes, and shone lights into my eyes. He also tried several of the "don't let me move your arm" and "push against my hand," tests, which I failed miserably. I was embarrassed by my weak muscles. Even after a full month at physiotherapy, I could barely resist any pressure.

The doctor showed me the brain MRI that was taken immediately after the seizures and explained all the findings to me. It was fascinating to see a picture of my brain, but I didn't know what he was talking about as he pointed to various spots and went on about brain swelling using neurological jargon. I was told that he was going to book another MRI to make sure my brain had returned to normal and to start weaning myself off the anti-seizure medication. It had to be done at some point, but I don't think there would be any time that it wouldn't be terrifying. It was a gamble to see if the medication was keeping the seizures at bay or if it was indeed a one-time thing.

Most people post-transplant are able to return to driving after three months, but the neurologist didn't want me to drive until I had been off the medication and seizure-free for an additional three months, because there was a chance I could have another seizure. I understood the logic and didn't want to have a seizure behind the wheel, but it was hard to have Isaiah drive me everywhere. I enjoyed downtown city driving much more than he did.

On April 1, I had had enough lying around the apartment recovering. I had a day off from hospital appointments and physiotherapy, so I took the bike we had borrowed for a short ride—emphasis on *short*. Nonetheless, it was an actual bike ride outside on an actual bike. I only made it around the small park before my body started madly protesting, but this was still more cycling than I had done in over a year. (I didn't consider using the exercise bike to be actual cycling.)

The ride was rejuvenating for me, both physically and emotionally. I remembered how much I loved cycling and then got emotional that it had been so long. It made me realize that even though I had lived in Toronto for a year and a half, I hadn't explored the immediate area where we lived. I always went to other neighbourhoods to visit when they were having festivals or parades. I never had the energy to go exploring just for the fun of it. When I realized that I now had the chance, it was liberating. In that moment, I felt immensely grateful to my donor.

⚜

The big question after being discharged from the hospital was this: when would I be cleared to move back to the Maritimes? The Almighty Transplant Manual said that everyone post-transplant has physiotherapy and weekly clinic appointments for the first three months. After three months, the team refers people to their local physiotherapists or sends them off into the wilderness. However, due to my lengthy hospital stay and frequent infections, no one would give me a clear answer as to when they thought all of my complications would be sorted and I would be able to return to Nova Scotia. I kept hearing, "Well, not this week," as though I would be prepared to move back on a week's notice. It wouldn't have mattered when I was officially discharged from their program, except that we needed to give two months' notice on the apartment. I didn't particularly want to end up paying rent for an extra two months or give notice too early and end up living in a family member's basement.

Eventually, I was told to expect to be in Toronto until at least my six-month testing, which gave me a better timeline. With that information and my desire to have a structured weekly artistic activity, I signed up again for a pottery class. I debated with myself and Isaiah about whether or not I should sign up for the eight-week session, but I figured it was my emotional therapy and worth the risk of being discharged early.

I continued to build strength at physiotherapy and finally made it back to my pre-transplant speed and elevation on the treadmill. My legs were screaming, but I barely coughed. Although I kept hoping that I would be able to fly past my old numbers, that didn't happen. My body struggled for a long time to do anything faster than a brisk walk. I stumbled over my feet whenever I attempted to jog to catch the bus. I hadn't expected to be able to sprint around town, but because I could make a short push to catch a bus pre-transplant, I thought I should still be able to do so post-transplant. As it happened, jogging was one of the last muscle memory activities to return.

During my physical recovery, I started having trouble with my left knee: my old cycling injury had returned with a vengeance, and it took an even longer time to strengthen the weak point in my legs. The physiotherapists told me to take a break from cycling and to rest it whenever possible. It helped but I wasn't good at the resting part. I finally had energy and I wanted to use it, dammit. All the physical improvement helped my lung function, which slowly improved as my lungs strengthened and I found I had more energy during the day. I didn't notice a change from day-to-day, but when I charted out my numbers from the month, it was encouraging to see a 0.5L improvement of my FEV1.

The second week of April, I had my second MRI to see if my brain had returned to normal, post-seizures. It had! Another highlight of the month was getting rid of the oxygen equipment. After my previous bronchoscopy, the doctor gave me the okay to cancel my home oxygen. I was given a discontinued prescription, called VitalAire, and they sent someone to pick up the equipment that had been gathering dust over the last three months. It was cathartic to get rid of that constant reminder of being sick. It was also great to free up some room in our tiny condo.

By mid-April, I was officially discharged from physiotherapy. The physiotherapists decided that my progress was good enough that I was ready to be on my own. Now when I exercised on a treadmill it would no longer be considered *physiotherapy* and would simply be *exercising*. As part of the discharge spiel, I was told that each week I should aim for at least 150 minutes of aerobic exercise, two days of weight training, and two days of good full-body stretching. At first I was concerned that I wouldn't be able to motivate myself to exercise that frequently, but I soon realized that it wouldn't be a problem.

My five-month post-transplant mark was fabulous. I managed to get a FEV1 of 1.78, which was my highest yet. I went for a celebratory bike ride in the morning since it was so beautiful outside. I still had to bundle up as I got cold quickly, but it was worth it. It still felt remarkable any time I was able to go for a long walk or bike ride. I had a hard time realizing that it was possible to do those activities without having a coughing fit or draining my energy for three days.

One of my fears before the transplant was that I would have the surgery and then spend all of my time afterward either hospitalized or in appointments at the hospital. For the first three months, it seemed like that fear was coming true. After spending the first two months in the hospital, once I was finally discharged, it seemed like I was still spending all of my time and energy at or waiting for appointments. I was starting to feel as though I endured the surgery just to live at the hospital. April 2015 was when that started to change. There were fewer appointments and being discharged from physiotherapy also significantly cut back my hospital time. I still had to go to the hospital two or three times a week for blood work, but it was no longer a twenty-hour a week commitment. I was finally able to spend my energy on activities I enjoyed, which was a brilliant change. Of course, it helped that I had more energy and just felt better overall. Much to Isaiah's delight, I had more energy to cook and help out around the apartment. Also, much to his dismay, this meant I also started making a mad list of sightseeing I wanted to do before we left Toronto.

Two weeks into my self-motivation exercise regime, everything was going as smoothly as possible. I loved the fact that I had energy to be as active as I wanted and no longer had to calculate which one activity deserved my energy that day. Having a gym in the condo building was a boon: all I had to do every morning was take the elevator downstairs to exercise. Also, the fact that I had spent the previous year and a half exercising every Monday, Wednesday, and Friday conditioned me to keep going.

I soon realized that I didn't have to figure out a behavioural reinforcement system for myself. As cheesy as it sounds, I was so excited I could do all these activities again that being able to bike ten kilometres without much struggle was rewarding on its own. I got up in the morning and wanted to go to the gym or out for a walk simply because I could, and I loved feeling how much stronger my body was getting. I also loved that my jeans were no longer falling off me as my legs strengthened and I gained weight. The fact that I was finally progressing quickly felt incredible and kept me motivated to keep going.

The downside to the exercising was that my knee pain kicked into high gear. I had injured my knee while cycling across Canada, and the injury returns to haunt me every once in a while. I ignored it for a week, hoping it would somehow resolve itself, but as it didn't, I had to start wrapping, icing, and resting it. I optimistically tried to start jogging very, very slowly, which went well and I felt great, until my knee gave out on me two days later. Then I could barely walk. In my joy of being able to once again run, I had started too quickly even though I thought

I was going slowly. My body wasn't ready for what my brain wanted me to be able to do. To this day, my knee still flares up from time to time when I do too much and forget to wrap or ice it afterward.

On the advice of the medical team, Isaiah and I gave our two months' notice for the apartment at the end of April. We started crossing off our "see before we move" list, and most of the activities involved walking. We spent a big day at the zoo, where we saw every exhibit for the first time. We had visited the zoo a few times, but during the previous visits I had stuck to the main pavilions to reduce the amount of walking. This time we walked the entire thing and even went down the excruciatingly long hill to the Canadian exhibit to see the bears, bison, and raccoons. Oh, my! I still find it funny that they had a raccoon in the zoo as it seems there is a raccoon living at the bottom of just about every garbage can in Toronto.

We also started walking home from hospital appointments every once in a while, through the markets, and I went for longer and longer bike rides along the waterfront. The waterfront trail was perfect for me to get back into biking. It was paved and off the road so I didn't have to worry about cars; best of all, it was almost completely flat. The downside was that it was always windy. One low point was when I had a jogger pass me while I struggled to get down the trail. My legs were still weak and a headwind only impeded my progress. The fact that a jogger passed me made me feel even weaker. I kept reminding myself that the jogger was probably not recovering from major surgery and that it was okay to be moving slowly—at least I was moving. I repeated that mantra a lot during the recovery phase.

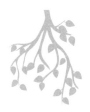

21

SIX MONTHS OF BEING ALIVE

At the end of May I had my six-month assessment and was told I would be officially discharged sometime in June. I was six months post-transplant and feeling wonderful.

I had another bronchoscopy, for which I was absolutely terrified. I panicked before we left the house, and again in the waiting room, and again in the freezing room. Isaiah did his best to reassure me that it couldn't possibly go worse than the other times. I relayed my fears to the doctor and she must have taken me seriously because soon after getting the sedative, I woke up in the recovery room. It still wasn't pleasant but at least I didn't remember most of it and didn't have the "I'm choking and about to die" sensation. My chart was already prepped with a comment about my near faints so they kept me longer and sent me off in a wheelchair just to be extra safe that I wouldn't collapse. And I didn't. It was, after all, significantly better than the previous times.

I had my major appointments the next day. An already long hospital day proved doubly long as the computers were running slowly in the entire hospital and no one knew what to do. My results were about the same as the previous month: my PFTS were good, my x-ray and CT scan were clear, my wound was healing, and I was told my PICC line could be removed as soon as my bronch results came back negative.

We only had a month left in the city. My pottery class ended, and while I still managed to go to a few of the drop-in classes in June, my three-hour class and no waiting in line days were over. I was sad that pottery was finished, not just because I always have more ideas of fun objects to make, but because it was the end of a chapter. I was pleased that this chapter was closing, but I would miss the class and the people I had met there. Things are never black and white, and while leaving Toronto was good because it meant I had had a successful transplant, it was also sad because we liked the city and everything it had to offer.

The first week of June had significant steps in store. My bronchoscopy results were negative for infection and rejection, meaning that my PICC line could finally be removed. I didn't mind having the PICC line in, as it meant I didn't have to be poked when I needed blood work, but as it was getting warmer and I wanted to go swimming, I was okay with removing it. It also increased my risk of infection and clots, and worst of all, it made showering difficult because I had to wrap my arm so no water got on the line.

The doctor who pulled the PICC out was the same one I had seen during my days at St. Michael's. He was finishing his residency at the end of June, just in time for me to leave. It was serendipitous how his residency followed my lung transplant timeline, first at St. Michael's, then pre-transplant at Toronto General, then ICU, then in-patient, and finally the outpatient clinics. Thanks for always being there for me, doc!

The other big step was that my wound finally healed over. After five months, all it had left to show for itself was a giant scar and a slightly smaller sternum. Before the wound got infected and I needed surgery, almost every nurse told me how great my incision looked and how the cut would heal quickly and I wouldn't have much of a scar. Unfortunately, because of the infection and subsequent surgery, that dream didn't last long. The wound area, which wasn't much of a wound by the end, turned into a giant mass of scar tissue and I still don't have full feeling on my left side in that area. I was officially discharged from homecare—no more having to wait around for nurses to show up—and I could finally shower whenever I wanted.

As soon as the hole from my PICC line healed over, I went for a swim in the condo pool. Chlorine water has never felt so good. I managed to do a few laps before I ran out of energy, but it was exhilarating to be back in water and able to return to another activity I loved so much.

We spent the rest of the month visiting as much of Toronto as possible. Unfortunately, due to my poor knee I couldn't walk around as much as I had hoped. We visited the Toronto Islands a few times and eventually made it kayaking around the islands, which was fun. I made it to a few more pottery drop-in classes and visited my extended family in the area one last time. We began packing and sorting our possessions in preparation for our journey home.

Everyone kept asking me if I was excited to move back to Nova Scotia, and honestly, my feelings were mixed. I enjoyed living in Toronto, and while I always knew it wouldn't be a permanent move, I was sad to leave. It was different living there and being able to do everything versus when I couldn't do as much pre-transplant. I mean, I did as much as I could before the transplant, but now that I could do so much more, I kept thinking of all the activities we needed to try before we left. We saw a lot of the city, but there was always one more beach or festival or museum to visit. That is the great part about living in Toronto.

I would make comments like, "It's happened so fast."

Isaiah usually responded with, "Umm, no, it hasn't."

I didn't mean that the wait or transplant recovery was quick in any way; it just felt like we were leaving as soon as I was starting to feel great and ready to explore more of the city. I know that's how it's supposed to happen: clearly the government wasn't going to subsidize my rent for me to vacation in Toronto. They wanted me home as soon as possible.

Medically, I did feel ready to leave. I felt as though I finally had a handle on the medication and what to do if something went wrong. I had not been ready at the three-month mark when the team had briefly discussed the possibility of my discharge. I was just being my typical self, becoming nostalgic about leaving a place even if wasn't full of excellent memories. I did have some good memories of Toronto, but I also had some almost-died-not-so-great ones. The stress of moving also kicked in and made me think even more about how much easier it would be if we didn't have to pack.

The non-nostalgic part of me was excited to be heading back to the Maritimes. I couldn't wait to see my friends and family again and head off to the beach. I wanted to have a quiet space that gets dark at night without using a sleep mask. Although someone pointed out to me that I had actually lived in Toronto longer than I had in Springhill, I still continued to refer to Springhill as home. Toronto was always a temporary home. I think because we saw it as such, we did as much as we could in the time we were there—that is partly why we enjoyed it so much.

On June 26, 2015, exactly seven months since my transplant and about twenty-one months since moving to Toronto, we loaded up our car to the bursting point and headed home: Springhill, Nova Scotia.

CURVEBALL

THE BIG C

That was supposed to be the end of the book. I was going summarize my story with descriptions of how we moved back to the Maritimes, had a beautiful summer of travelling around to visit family (to see them and collect our stored possessions), spent days on the beach, and went on long hikes. And we did all that; it was incredible. I was going to go on about the wonders of feeling better than I had in years and how amazing it was that I could return to my favourite pastimes again. Every activity I was able to resume caused me to cry with elation; there were a lot of happy tears that summer. Everything was going smoothly and life seemed to be stabilizing. I was getting blood work done every other week and PFTs monthly (I still do them every morning with my micro spirometer). I was astounded at how much energy I had. The family booked a celebration trip to Aruba for November so we could all get away to celebrate my transplant. I was excited to be able to travel once again. I've mentioned my love of travelling, and booking the trip made me feel like I was starting to be able to return to everything that I loved.

But then, in August 2015, I started coughing. My lung function dropped a bit, and I felt more tired than usual. I called the clinic to inform them. The doctors figured it was just a cold, so I got some antibiotics, was put on aerosol masks, and didn't think much of it. I headed to Toronto at the end of August for my nine-month assessment. The assessment went smoothly overall, even with my waking up at the end of my bronchoscopy. Unfortunately though, the results from the bronchoscopy showed that I had an infection in my lungs.

The infection didn't seem like a big deal, but it did explain why I wasn't feeling the best. I began new medication so when I started getting light-headed while exercising and my hemoglobin dropped, I, and the doctors, wrote it off as just adjusting to the new drugs. However, I never seemed to improve. When my levels dropped low enough that I needed a blood transfusion at the start of October, I started to think it was more than a reaction to medication.

The doctors wanted to investigate further, so I went in for a bronchoscopy in Halifax at the end of October. I got a fever afterward, and as a result, was immediately hospitalized. That's when the doctors started a full-on investigation to find out why my hemoglobin continued to drop. I kept reminding them that I needed to be out by November 13 because I was off to Aruba, and they couldn't stop me.

Well, they figured out a way to stop me. After massive amounts of blood work, a couple of CT scans, and a liver and bone marrow biopsy, on Friday, November 13, I was told I had post-transplant lymphoproliferative disorder (PTLD). The big C. The one I had been warned about before my transplant that I had all but ignored because the chances of getting it were 5–10%. I was devastated. At that moment, I was more frustrated that I was sitting in the hospital instead of boarding a plane to sunny Aruba with the rest of my family than I was concerned about the cancer. This wasn't the grand post-transplant life that I had been promised. (Okay, so no one ever promised me anything, but I felt like they should've.) I had survived the transplant and now I had to deal with cancer? It didn't seem fair. The full implications of having cancer wouldn't hit until I was transferred to the hematology unit at Halifax's Victoria General (VG) hospital, now a site of the QEII Health Sciences Centre, and started chemotherapy.

The months of waiting and being in and out of the hospital so frequently before my transplant had made me fluent in the language of "hospitalese." I had been well-versed before, but the transplant solidified my fluency. It's a language you learn to be able to answer questions about your life in thirty seconds: "No I don't smoke, no recreational drugs, maybe one alcoholic drink a week, my blood pressure usually runs low, and here is my list of medication." You learn what BID (two times a day), NPO (nothing by mouth), CBC (complete blood count) mean, and that the LPNS (licensed practical nurses) won't touch a PICC line unless it's to help wrap it for the shower. No one wants to become comfortable in hospitals, but the faster you can learn the language, the easier it is to navigate the system.

I think part of the shock of being diagnosed with cancer was that I had to learn an entirely new language, the language of cancer. It did help that I was used to the hospital system so at least I was accustomed to having a nurse shine a flashlight in my eyes at 2:00 A.M. or being wakened with a cold breakfast at 7:00 A.M. Even so, there was still a huge adjustment to the new diagnosis and everything that came with it. I did what everyone tells you *not* to do and went to Dr. Internet to look up my diagnosis, common treatments, and predicted outcomes. It actually helped me because I learned more than what the doctors had told me. Or more realistically, what the doctor had probably told me, but after she said, "You have post-transplant lymphoproliferative disease," I forgot everything else she said. (I recommend everyone take a companion when getting test results because it's hard to hear anything or ask questions after being told yours are positive. And if everything is negative, there is someone to enjoy a "good news" celebratory coffee with.)

I was transferred from the general admission floor to the specialized hematology floor at Halifax's VG site with its tiny rooms. There they recommended not drinking the water or showering due to the risk of legionnaires' disease, and when I was there, they were recovering from a flood after some pipes had burst. I was introduced to the team who would be taking over my care, and while they were all lovely, there was also an acclimatization period with new health-care professionals. I had felt immediately comfortable with the CF team in Toronto, probably because the staff didn't rotate as much as the transplant team so I came to know each doctor better. The months that I spent waiting had helped me trust that they were doing all they could during my two months of steady decline. I love my Halifax respiratory team and have such a good rapport with them that it was difficult to relay all my concerns to the new cancer health-care team. With the addition of another team caring for me, I wasn't sure which doctor was in charge when someone told me about a medication change. It was an adjustment period, learning the new system and the different hospital.

I managed to get a bed in the Bone and Marrow Transplant wing of the hematology floor, which in comparison was the Ritz. The room was large with enough chairs for multiple visitors, modern cupboards, and a decent-sized bathroom. However, I was back in the world of inspirational phrases and terrible metaphors: I was the umbrella in the storm of my life and the rainbow after the storm was hope. Who comes up with these sayings? I don't have a problem with people trying to cheer up a room, especially when bone marrow transplant patients spend months in the hospital, but there is nothing wrong with a pretty painting with no metaphors.

The inspirational quotes must help some people, but I didn't understand how they were supposed to help me. I need ones that say, "Just get through this," "Grit your teeth and bear it," or, "Life can be terrible and random; accept it and move on." There was no silver lining to getting cancer. It was terrible. It didn't make me a better person, see the world as a better place, or appreciate every day as a blessing. I think almost dying from lung failure had that part sewn up. I don't need a quote telling me to try to find the positive angle. I'm a firm believer that not every situation has to teach you a lesson and not everything that happens in life has to be defining or rewarding. Sometimes events happen that are simply random and terrible and it's enough to get through it without learning anything. It's okay to just let bad times be bad times. I don't need to turn it into a life lesson.

Apart from feeling short of breath and faint when I exercised, I didn't feel sick in the way that I had leading up to my transplant. The chemotherapy made me quite ill but I always expected that I would recover from the cancer, even though the doctor told me how aggressively the cancer was moving. I'm not sure if it was arrogance or faith in the medical system, but some part of me thought that if I made it through the transplant, surely cancer couldn't kill me—of course, that's absurd and cancer can kill anyone. Or maybe I was just feeling more prepared since I had been through a death scare before. I think wrestling with all the death questions leading up to my transplant helped me emotionally when I received the cancer diagnosis. While the process was different from lung failure and I had some moments of feeling like I might actually die from this, I didn't have the panic that struck when my lungs first started to fail. I did update my funeral plan, but beyond that, I didn't have that immediate feeling that I had to seek out information.

I think it also made a difference that I was already in the hospital when I was diagnosed and was started on treatment immediately. I didn't have much time to think about the broader picture of dying. There was more a focus on just getting through the treatment and then seeing what would happen after that, whereas throughout the lung transplant process, I was often waiting around, so I had plenty of time to think about dying. While I felt relatively fine before chemotherapy started, I knew that my diagnosis was serious when almost every doctor and nurse asked me about a POA. No one had asked me about it so often as during that first cancer hospitalization. It reinforced how serious my diagnosis was and how quickly they would have to respond. I know the team just wanted to make sure I was covered if something went wrong, but the frequent questions about my end-of-life plan did not match the hopeful vibe I was going for.

Before my first chemotherapy infusion, I was supposed to have "chemotherapy training," but since I was an in-patient, a pharmacist and doctor visited my room to tell me about all the terrible side effects. I was told that 95% of people on the same chemotherapy medication as me lost their hair in the first six to eight weeks, that I could get some numbness in my fingers and toes, that my blood sugars would spike, and then all about the usual fatigue, nausea, and diarrhea side effects. After they left, the pharmacist ran back in to tell me, "Oh, by the way, there is a good chance these medications will make you sterile."

I asked if she could guarantee that, since it would save on birth control in the future. I was fine with casually being told I would be unable to have children. I had never wanted kids so it wasn't devastating news, although I can imagine it would be for a lot of women. There wasn't any time to harvest and save eggs if I had wanted to because chemotherapy started a few hours after that visit.

Some women with CF have children, but the risks tend to be high. It's also hard to get pregnant because the extra mucous that grows in the lungs is also in the uterus. And once a woman is pregnant, the extra calories required can be difficult to maintain. Further in the pregnancy, the fetus tends to press on the lungs which can make breathing even more difficult. All in all, it's a high-risk decision. I decided long ago that the risk wasn't worth it for me. There is also the fact of having a short life expectancy, which would leave the partner as a single parent at some point. I respect the women who have made that decision for their families, but I never pictured it for myself. In any case, now if there was even a sliver of doubt that I might someday have children, it was taken away.

A few hours later, the nurses came in with full protection gear and hooked up the first chemotherapy drug to my IV. I was getting the full R-CHOP treatment, which is five different medications, four of them transfused via IV in about six hours. The first time was longer because they had to make sure I wouldn't react to the drug (I didn't). The medication was painless. All I had to think about was when I would be discharged from the hospital. I made it home before Christmas but was back in on my twenty-ninth birthday with what would become my usual fever week.

Generally, people tend to get PTLD in one location, and it's treated with a once-a-week dosage of a drug called Rituximab for four weeks. However, on my investigative PET scan (formally, positron emission tomography scan), it showed that there was lymphoma in my liver, lungs, spleen, and various other parts of the body. The cancer was moving quickly so the doctors had to react just as aggressively. The survival rates for PTLD are about 55% after five years; however, the hematologist told me to take that number with a giant grain of salt because it covers all transplants, not just lung. She said it included the elderly men who got kidney transplants and may have died from complications other than the cancer.

When I was discharged from the hospital in Toronto I had decided I would continue to let my hair grow out since, in all my time recovering, it had surpassed the awkward "growing out" stage. It's true what they say about the best laid plans often going awry. It was a year later, when my hair was almost shoulder-length, that the pharmacist told me the majority of women lose their hair with the treatment I was having, so I should plan for it to fall out six to eight weeks after my first chemotherapy dose.

After my first dose of chemotherapy, I decided that since my hair was going to fall out in a month, I should dye it a fun colour before saying goodbye. I was still in the hospital, and one of my friends agreed to help me. We both put on the terrible yellow isolation protective gowns and got to work, first bleaching, then dyeing my hair. The nurses didn't mind the mess too much—purple dye was everywhere—and helpfully brought us towels. I'm sure the laundry staff were baffled by the purple towels. It was so much fun. However, as she was rinsing the dye out of my hair, it started to fall out. It was only one week after my first dose of chemotherapy. It didn't fall out in dramatic clumps, but it was enough to freak me out. The next day the hair loss was worse, so I stopped touching my head as much as possible in hopes that would keep my hair attached. Of course, that was a ridiculous notion. Another friend stopped by with her razor and gave me a trendy undercut to help me deal with the hair loss. The purple look didn't last long.

I didn't think I would be part of the 5% of people who keep their hair, but I did think I had longer than a week. I hadn't even ordered a wig at that point. Having hair fall out every time I touched my head and waking up with hair all over my pillow was traumatizing. I knew I could handle the being bald part, although that did take some adjusting. I've had short pixie cuts in the past, so it wasn't as much of a shock for me as it would be for someone who has had long hair their entire life. The worst part was having it fall out slowly, day after day, and holding handfuls of hair every time I washed it. That was disturbing. Moments like that should be left to horror films and not happen in real life.

Once I was discharged from the hospital, a week before Christmas, I went to the barber and had him buzz the rest of my head. It felt better, emotionally, to be taking control of the situation. I still lost all the short hairs that hung on for a few weeks, but it wasn't as noticeable and was significantly less upsetting than waking up in the morning with long hair on my pillow. I eventually ordered two wigs (wig shopping was surprisingly fun—there are so many interesting options on Etsy) and was gifted two more. I became proficient at wrapping my head in scarves, and since it was winter, I mostly just wore toques. As the weeks went on, my scalp became tender and I found I had to wear a nightcap so it wouldn't be irritated by the pillow. I also switched to using baking soda and diluted apple cider vinegar as shampoo. It was like a science experiment on my head.

Once I had lost all my hair (except a few stubborn eyebrow hairs that managed to be stronger than chemotherapy), I managed okay. I became proficient at filling in my eyebrows and using eyeliner to hide the fact that I had no eyelashes. It's odd that at a time when I could not have felt less feminine, I experimented more with makeup and earrings than I ever had before. I wouldn't call it freeing because it was still hard to deal with, but it wasn't the traumatic experience I thought it might be. That's not to say that I wasn't self-conscious about being completely bald—I was. I didn't like not having something on my head while out in public, but it wasn't something that I worried about all the time. I think the fact that most of my experience happened during the winter helped; toques were soft for my tender scalp and kept me warm. When I did start wearing wigs, it wasn't too hot out. As it warmed up, I found the wigs became hot to deal with, but at that point my hair was starting to grow back, so I embraced the Furiosa look.

I didn't even notice that my hair was growing back until a friend pointed it out. I was only on round six of chemotherapy at that point so I didn't expect that it would return until I was finished treatment. But I was wrong. It grew back slowly, and thankfully not in patches or thinly as it does for some people. The doctor warned me that it would return curly. And it did. I've always had wavy hair, but growing up, my brother was the only one in the family with perfect ringlets when he let his hair grow out as a rebellious teenager. Not anymore. Apparently one of the random side effects from some chemotherapy medication is changing the hair follicles so they tend to grow back curly for the first year and may then relax some. The only surprising part was the amount of grey in my hair. Clearly, medical trauma turns you grey.

The winter of my cancer treatment we spent a lot of time driving back and forth to Halifax. (I say we drove, when in fact Isaiah drove while I napped.) I had my chemotherapy infusion and an intrathecal injection and then would return home to lie in bed for two days as required to not get headaches from the movement of my spinal fluid. The injections were one of the most painful parts of cancer. As any woman who has had an epidural knows, having a giant needle jabbed into the spine is terrible. Like most procedures, the freezing needle (or needles, depending on the competency of the doctor) was the worst part.

After I recovered from the intrathecal injections, I would have a few good days when I tried to get outside or do something active. The good days decreased as the accumulation of the medication in my system intensified.

I had to give myself white cell booster needles for the ten days following chemotherapy. The injections burned while being administered and had painful side effects, but the daily needle did cure my fear of self-injection. I was offered homecare services but I didn't want to wait around for the nurse every day for an injection, so I suggested to the team that Isaiah could do it. After yelling at Isaiah for a few days because he pushed the dose in too fast, I decided it would be better if I did it myself. It was a hard psychological boundary to cross; however, I felt much better once I was able to do it on my own.

Even with the white cell boosters, every chemotherapy cycle my white cell count (the cells of the immune system that fight off infection) would drop so dangerously low that I would get a fever, requiring hospitalization. The first few cycles I stayed in my hometown because I didn't know that I was going to get a fever every time. However, after one visit, the smaller hospitals didn't want to touch me, so they shipped me off to Halifax as soon as they could, where I would be with the specialized doctors. We drove to Halifax at the end of the first week and stayed at a friend's house to wait because it was easier to be admitted through the Halifax emergency department than going through the rural hospitals first.

Waiting for the fever was terrible. I tried to have everything prepared and a bag packed for the hospital, but at first it was just a waiting game. After several cycles, I knew it would hit at exactly the seventh night, until it moved to the sixth night, taking me by surprise. I never got any sleep those nights. The white cell booster had the side effect of making me feel as though the bones in my legs were growing and also like someone had punched me in the jaw. The pain medication they gave me didn't help much. Then the fever would hit and I would be incapacitated. Isaiah would have to practically carry me out of bed and to the car while I tried not to pass out or throw up. I would be so cold that I would shake uncontrollably, and nothing except medication and time would help. I never had to wait long in the emergency department before I got a room and was wrapped in as many hot blankets as possible.

The fear of pain is something that people talk about before they get a transplant, but I was fine following mine. I was on a lot of medication that kept me calm and allowed me to move around as much as possible. There was discomfort around some of the stitches, but I never felt the sharp, unyielding pain I experienced with chemotherapy. I'm sure I was on much stronger medication post-transplant than they gave me during chemotherapy, but the pain was also different. The pain after transplant was more of an extended ache, while the side effect pain I had from the white cell booster injections was a stabbing bone pain. Without exaggeration, I can say it was the worst pain of my life.

The Halifax emergency team was generally great, except the few times when a resident would want to review my life story while I was sleeping or a doctor wanted to insert a catheter for reasons I still don't understand. After I was stable I would eventually be transferred to the hematology floor where I would be hydrated, given antibiotics (due to the fear of an infection), have my blood replenished, and sleep for a few days. When my white cell count was in less critical range, I was sent home to recover for my next cycle. It was terrible.

During those few days in the hospital, I would often have panic attacks from the pain or lack of sleep. I had to keep repeating to myself what the nurse told me during my transplant panic attacks the previous year: they would only last fifteen minutes—fifteen minutes of high stress and hyperventilating. I would ask the nurses for more pain medication or a sedative, but those often took a while to kick in, leaving me ample time to panic. I have no other way to describe it than to say that my brain would lie to me. I would feel worthless and would wonder if life was worth living. I wasn't suicidal but I did feel unbelievably sad. In those moments, I would feel like all the pain wasn't worth it and I wanted to quit treatment. It's scary how fast the transition would be from feeling normal to feeling hopeless. It took some time for me to recognize that it was the medication messing with my brain and then I would feel fine the next day. But during those times, it was real. I would call either Amy or Isaiah and rant on the phone for a while until I felt better or fell asleep. It was unfortunate that the panic attacks tended to happen at 3:00 A.M., when I couldn't sleep from the pain.

When I was admitted during my chemotherapy fevers, I spent the majority of my time reading. I went through many books (shout out to libraries and their massive collections of e-books). I read Susan Mallery, Eloisa James, and Michael Connelly. I also read books from my childhood like the Harry Potter series and David Eddings's works, books that were familiar and made me feel like I was wrapped in a comforting blanket. (Sometimes I would watch Netflix on my computer, but because the hospital internet was unreliable, this was often more frustration than it was worth.) The romance stories about a woman who recently got dumped, or whose dog died, or who lost her job, or all three, before finding the perfect guy, never failed to keep my attention. It helped that I could predict the ending from the first page. Over the years I've discovered that hospital books shouldn't be more complicated than ones that ask, "How will they get together?" or "Who killed that person?"

After eight intensive rounds of R-CHOP chemotherapy with intrathecal injections, I had another PET scan that showed the pain was worth it. I had made it through. I'm now considered to be in remission with a "low chance of recurrence," according to my hematologist. Recovering from the effects of the chemotherapy medication took many months, although it was hard to know when recovery ended because there was no quick transformation. It was a slow build: my appetite and energy would increase slightly each week. I gained the weight back that I had lost and began exercising in earnest again. There is not much positive I can say about having CF, but one of the few benefits is that it has given me an ability to push my body to its limits. I think that helped speed up my recovery as I cycled and hiked around my area of the world.

Isaiah's and my relationship had to go through a similar transition as it had following the transplant. While I had chemotherapy, Isaiah was once more thrust into the caregiver role. The cancer was different because my energy levels were so cyclical, depending on where I was in the chemotherapy cycle. I wouldn't be able to move the day after chemo due to the intrathecal injections, so Isaiah would have to bring me food while I lay in bed and complained. I would then feel okay until the fever hit a week later. Then he would have to drag me out of bed and to the hospital, otherwise I would've stayed curled into a ball under the blankets. The one thing that may have eased the caregiver role slightly during chemotherapy was that I was in the hospital for my worst days. He didn't have to take care of me because the hospital was doing that. Instead, he was required to bring me coffee and watermelon (I had such watermelon cravings during chemotherapy), although he also got the 3:00 A.M. phone calls when I was having panic attacks.

I think it helps that Isaiah knows where the boundaries are and when I actually need support. After so much time together and a lot of communication, we have a good system. He generally knows when to leave me alone and when I want someone around. My first night on the hematology floor the nurse asked Isaiah if he wanted a cot set up so he could spend the night. He gave her a funny look and laughed as though he didn't know why he would ever want to sleep at the hospital. At that point, I had spent so many nights in the hospital that having someone stay with me would be more of a stressor than anything. There was no point in both of us being tired and grumpy from lack of sleep.

The seemingly continuous attempt of my body to die is not always easy on my relationship with Isaiah, but I think it did give us perspective in the long run. I would like to say that we don't fight over the small potatoes and we appreciate each other all the time, but that's not how life is. We still squabble because that's how our relationship functions. His clothes on the floor still annoy me and my earrings all over the house annoy him, but I don't think there is ever any avoiding those parts of a relationship. Most importantly, we know we can get through the "sickness" part of a relationship.

By the end of that summer, I was feeling ready to go on a short trip outside of the Maritimes. Before my transplant, when I couldn't walk to the bus stop without getting short of breath or having a coughing fit, I said the one thing I wanted to do if I got new lungs was to hike Gros Morne Mountain in Newfoundland. It was the only real concrete goal I set for myself. At the time, it was hard to imagine I would be able to walk more than a block comfortably, let alone hike up a mountain.

Gros Morne may seem random as there are many beautiful hikes around the Maritimes. However, it was one that I had been close to doing several times but had never been physically able to handle. The first time was when we visited as a family in the '90s. Mom and Dad weren't sure how hard the hike would be and figured that David and I were too young, so we stayed behind with Mom and went to the Rocky Harbour pool while Amy and Dad did the trek.

Then, years later, when David and I finished cycling across Canada, and Mom and Dad drove over to St. John's to pick us up, we took a family vacation around the island, including Gros Morne National Park. I was much too exhausted to do anything more than a few short hikes and look for whales, so I stayed behind at camp with Isaiah while David, Mom, and Dad went up the mountain.

Finally, when Amy and I visited The Rock and I got short of breath while doing the short Tablelands hike, I knew there was no way I could hike up Gros Morne. We didn't even consider it. The mountain had always eluded me, but now I finally felt ready to tackle it. My family, never ones to be left behind for a vacation, planned the trip. All five of us (Mom, Dad, Amy, Isaiah, and I) loaded into Mom and Dad's small hatchback with our camping gear and off we went.

The weather on the day of our hike couldn't have been better. It was cool and cloudy, which was perfect for the steep climb. I was excited once we got to the trail and felt like I would fly right up. Amy, to no one's surprise, decided to hike too, with her oxygen tank in a backpack. (As of writing, Amy now requires oxygen "upon exertion" and remains in that limbo-land where her lung function is too high to be eligible for a transplant but too low to be able to continue working as a nurse. It's a weird role reversal where, for once, I am the healthier one watching my sister's health decline.)

Amy started the hike by saying that she would just walk to the base and "see how she felt" before deciding whether she would do the entire thing. The four kilometres to the base, mostly on an incline, were a struggle for her. It was early morning so there was a lot of coughing, throwing up, and many breaks. She kept going and pushed through what looked like a desire to curl into a ball by the side of the trail to have a nap.

When we got to the base, the mountain had cleared but it was still cloudy and cool, with no humidity. It was a perfect day for reaching the summit. Amy decided to keep going with us because, while her lungs weren't happy, she wasn't experiencing the jabbing pain that sometimes occurs—although I'm not sure what would've turned her back at that point. We took many breaks and seemed to be passed by almost everyone, though somehow (I think through determination and a competitive spirit) Amy and the rest of us made it to the top.

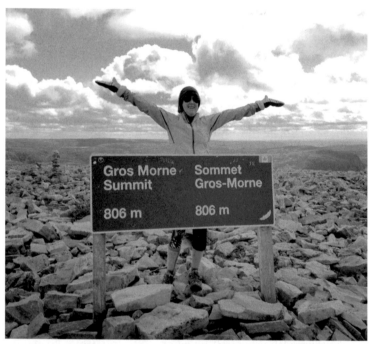

Allison had a hard time imagining life post-transplant—but her one goal, if the surgery was a success, was to hike Gros Morne Mountain in Newfoundland. In 2016, she triumphantly reached the summit. (Donna Watson)

I can't fully articulate how I felt at the top. I was so thrilled and excited to have made it. It signified more than just a hike to all of the family. The man who took our picture said, "It's a struggle up, isn't it?" To which Mom mumbled, "More than you know." And that sums it up: I had finally bounced back from years of illness, from not being able to climb stairs without coughing, to being able to summit mountains.

The accomplishment was more psychological than anything else. Sure, the hike wasn't a stroll in the park, but it wasn't intensely hard. It was no more exhausting than the two days of the Fundy Circuit I had done a month prior. It's not like anything had changed during that week or I had suddenly become significantly stronger. It's that I never truly believed I would have the chance to do it again. I was conquering mountains that I had dreamed of before my transplant.

I'm still not exactly sure how Amy made it through the hike with her low lung function. I think she wanted to see how far she could physically push herself. Because having CF is a constant struggle to stay healthy before you lose what health you have, testing physical limits seems to be par for the course. It's an attitude of, "Do what you can, when you can, because you never know if you'll ever be this healthy again." I'm sure not everyone feels this way, but Amy and I always push against our limitations as much as possible.

I still get a sense of awe when I can do everything I had only dreamed about before the transplant. As I've said, I was hesitant in agreeing to the lung transplant because it was a terrifying great unknown. I was scared to be hopeful for the future: I felt if I dreamed too much, it would only bring disappointment. It was also hard to dream about being able to hike, bike, and climb stairs without coughing when I didn't have much energy beyond day-to-day activities. In the end, post-transplant life is better than I could've dreamed, even though I had to overcome cancer. I sleep comfortably at night, I rarely cough, and I have the energy to wash dishes and climb mountains.

And all because someone agreed to be an organ donor. I am eternally grateful to the donor and their family. Without them, I would've died in the hospital. The team did everything they could to get the lungs to fit my body because they knew it was my only chance at survival. The lungs aren't the perfect fit, but that doesn't matter because I'm alive. Without years of research and funding, the scientific know-how of my doctors and entire health-care team, and most of all, the donor, I wouldn't be here today.

I do not know how long I have with my new lungs. There are no guarantees in this life. I may have a few more months, a year,

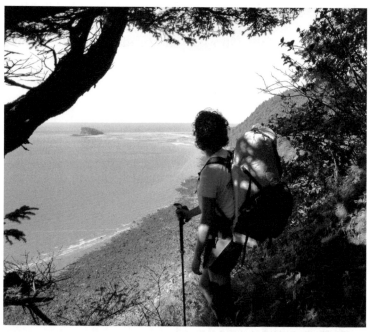

Before her transplant, Allison dreamed about having the energy to tackle major hikes. In 2018, she enjoyed a vigorous multi-day hike along the Fundy Footpath in New Brunswick. (Donna Watson)

or ten years. I don't know what the future holds, but I do know that whatever happens and whatever curveball comes my way, I am resilient and strong, and I can handle it.

AFTERWORD

I'm now just over four years post-transplant. My life is beyond what I could have imagined pre-transplant or during those months in recovery. I've participated in five-kilometre fun runs, I've started wilderness camping, and I feel physically strong. Because I live a relatively normal life, I sometimes forget that I don't have the same stamina as a normal healthy person. I still need to sleep a lot, avoid people who are sick because I pick up every germ, and it takes me longer than most people to recover from an infection. It's the reality of being immunocompromised and I've accepted it as part of my life, although sometimes I need to remind myself of that when I get frustrated with being tired or needing so much sleep.

My lungs remain stable, and I still go to Toronto every year around what I call my "lungiversary" to check in with the team and make sure I'm doing everything I should be. My hematology and transplant doctors have all said that the chance of cancer recurrence is low at this point, but I have an underlying fear it has returned every time I feel mysteriously dizzy or ill in

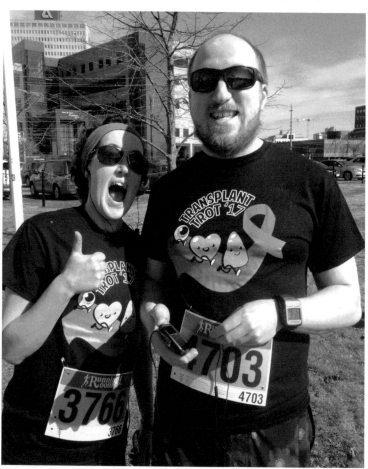

Allison and her partner, Isaiah, participated in the Transplant Trot in Moncton, NB, in April 2017. Allison has completed several five-kilometre fun runs post-transplant. (Amy Watson)

any way. I'm not sure the fear will ever completely subside, but much like rejection, every year it doesn't return means it's less likely to show up in the imminent future.

While I no longer have CF in my new lungs, I still have the pancreatic and digestive problems which cause issues from time to time. I get sickly dehydrated if I'm not careful, and I have to take extra precautions to avoid sunburns when I'm outside. I remain insulin-dependent, requiring multiple finger pokes to check my blood sugar levels and insulin injections a day. Being diabetic is the development that requires the most time and maintenance on a day-to-day basis.

In the past year, I was fortunate to attend a surf camp in Hawaii for young adults who had or have cancer. Everyone at the camp came from different parts of Canada and the United States and had a variety of cancers; they all had interesting stories. In between learning to surf and snorkelling with the sea turtles, we bonded over sharing medical stories, life experiences, and concerns for the future. It's rare that I'm able to physically meet people who have had similar experiences to mine, and I got more out of the opportunity than I had expected.

I've been fortunate to be able to travel elsewhere in the world. While trips around the Maritimes are fun, there's something about visiting a different country and experiencing a new culture that brings me immeasurable joy. The family had a redo of the "one-year lungiversary" celebration that I missed while in the hospital, only this time in Cuba. We relaxed, snorkelled, ate great food, and celebrated just being able to spend time together.

Although it was two years ago now, my thirtieth birthday—two years after my lung transplant, a year after my cancer diagnosis, and seven months since my last dose of chemotherapy—was one of the best birthdays of my life. This was not because of anything special I did that day; in fact, it was another regular Friday, only with cupcakes. However, the day still seemed like a milestone after everything I had been through. I had doubted so many times whether I would ever reach that point. Yet there I was, turning thirty, and I could not have been more excited. I had wondered many times if I would be alive to see it.

Every birthday that passes I'm reminded of how far I've come. I no longer feel my life is as defined by CF as I did during

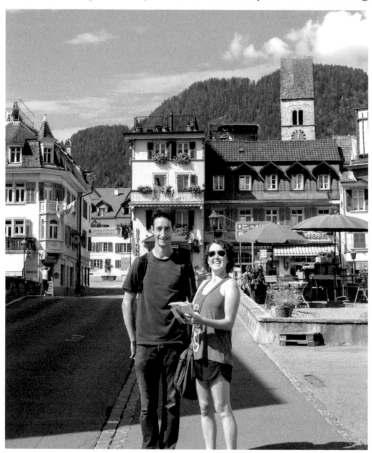

Since surviving a double-lung transplant and post-transplant lymphoproliferative disorder, a lymphoma-like form of cancer, Allison has enjoyed travelling to other parts of the world. She's seen here with her brother, David, in Switzerland in 2018. (Amy Watson)

my transplant years. I still have many medical appointments, but they have reduced over time as I remain stable. While I will always be on medication and require insulin, the daily medical care is now habitual, and I'm able to focus on and nurture other aspects of my life. I remain cautiously optimistic for the future and try to take advantage of opportunities that arise because I know too well that life is to be cherished.

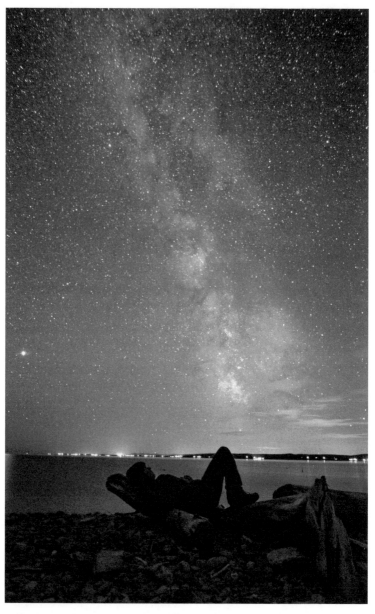

Allison gazes at the stars in Forillon National Park, Quebec, in 2018. (Amy Watson)

ACKNOWLEDGEMENTS

It's hard to believe what started as a collection of blog posts is now the much-condensed and coherent book you're holding. Many thanks to everyone who made this a reality: first and foremost, to those who read my blog and encouraged me to keep writing, thank you for following along. To those I sent a rough version of the book to, asking, "Do you think this is anything?" your feedback made me keep going. To my editor, Paula, for culling my adjective addiction. To Stefanie for doing the hard work of getting the book in working order so I could pitch it and not embarrass myself. To Melanie for being the most enthusiastic about everything I do and for always being there when I couldn't find the word I wanted.

To Jason and Heather, thank you for making our time in Toronto better. Between all the food you fed us, swims in the pool, and board games, you truly gave us a relaxing place to get away.

Thank you to everyone who wrote to me, brought me food, and played games with me while I was hospitalized, both in Halifax and Toronto. I couldn't have gotten through so well without you.

A million thanks to my parents for the clarification on parts of the family story and for not objecting when I said I wanted to publish a book about my life. Your support through everything has been immeasurable. To my siblings, thank you for the adventures and for responding to my late-night texts. And finally, to Isaiah, it's hard to describe how much your love and support have meant to me over the years. Thanks for sticking by me through it all.

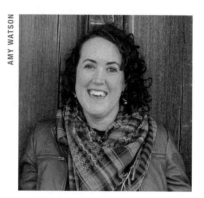

AMY WATSON

A LLISON WATSON BELIEVES IN LIVING every day to the fullest. Raised in Petitcodiac, New Brunswick, she had an active childhood despite daily treatment for cystic fibrosis. In 2014, she received new lungs in Toronto. As a side effect, she was diagnosed with post-transplant lymphoproliferative disorder. After intensive chemotherapy, she is now cancer free and is again able to physically do the things she enjoys. Allison Watson lives in Springhill, Nova Scotia.